Workbook for

Pharmacology for Pharmacy Technicians

Third Edition

Prepared by:

Anthony Guerra, M.HCI, PharmD, RPh
Professor, Chemistry/Pharmacology
Des Moines Area Community College
Ankeny, Iowa

ELSEVIER

ELSEVIER

3251 Riverport Lane
St. Louis, Missouri 63043

Publishing Director: Kristin Wilhelm
Senior Development Specialist: Laura Selkirk
Publishing Services Manager: Deepthi Unni
Project Manager: Nayagi Athmanathan

Printed in India

Last digit is the print number: 9 8 7 6 5 4 3

Preface

The goal of this workbook is to help students apply and master key concepts and skills presented in *Pharmacology for Pharmacy Technicians*, 3rd edition. The exercises in this workbook reinforce comprehension of material from the textbook.

The following exercises provide a sufficient review of concepts and allow students to apply the concepts from the text:

- Each chapter begins with a matching exercise of the **terms and definitions** in the text.
- **Fill-in-the-Blank** questions allow the student to review generic and brand name drugs.
- A variety of question formats test knowledge of concepts in the book, including **matching, multiple choice, and true/false**.

- **Critical thinking** exercises require students to use the knowledge they have learned in the chapter and apply it to specially designed exercises.
- **Research Activities** allow students to take the concepts they have learned and do additional research on various topics.
- **Case Studies** are designed to help students develop their analytical, critical thinking, and clinical reasoning skills. The case studies represent situations similiar to those the student may encounter in daily practice.

Best wishes as you begin your journey to become a pharmacy technician!

Table of Contents

1 Fundamentals of Pharmacology

TERMS AND DEFINITIONS

Match each term with the correct definition below.

A. Bioavailability
B. Biopharmaceuticals
C. Controlled substance
D. Dosage form
E. Dose
F. Dosing schedule
G. Drug
H. Drug delivery system
I. Enteral
J. Homeopathic medicines
K. Legend drug
L. Over-the-counter drug
M. Parenteral
N. Pharmacognosy
O. Pharmacology
P. Pharmacotherapy
Q. Toxicology

1. The study of the biological, biochemical features of drugs of plant and animal origins is called _____.

2. _____ is defined as the study of drugs and their interactions with living systems, including chemical and physical properties, toxicology, and therapeutics.

3. A(n) _____ is defined as a substance that is used to diagnose, treat, cure, prevent, or mitigate disease in humans or other animals.

4. A(n) _____ drug is administered orally, whereas a(n) _____ drug is administered by injection or infusion.

5. A(n) _____ may be obtained without a prescription, whereas _____ may be obtained only by prescription.

6. Medicines can be formulated into a different _____ (formulation) and a _____ is designed to release a specific amount of drug.

7. A drug may be classified as a(n) _____ to restrict its possession because of its potential for abuse.

8. The term used to describe the use of drugs for the treatment of disease is _____.

9. The _____ is the frequency that the drug is administered (e.g., "four times a day").

10. Drugs produced by the process of bioengineering involving recombinant DNA technology are classified as _____.

11. _____ is the science dealing with the study of poisons.

12. The term used to describe the extent to which a drug reaches the site of action and is available to produce its effects is _____.

13. _____ are drugs that are administered in minute quantities and that stimulate natural body healing systems.

14. If it is a _____, then it's the amount for just one application or administration.

MULTIPLE CHOICE

1. All of the following statements about pharmacy technicians who have a working knowledge of

   pharmacology are true *except* _____.
   A. pharmacy technicians' work performance will be more accurate and efficient.
   B. pharmacy technicians may be able to reduce dispensing errors.
   C. more time will be spent searching for drugs when pharmacy technicians have good brand/generic name recognition.
   D. the selection of appropriate warning labels (auxiliary labels) to place on prescription vials of dispensed medicines is made easier.
   E. pharmacy technicians understand the importance of alerting the pharmacy to drug interactions, therapeutic duplication, and excessive dose alerts screened by the computer.

2. Which Greek physician is considered to be the "father of pharmacology"?
   A. Dioscorides
   B. Theophrastus
   C. Emperor Shen Nung
   D. Hippocrates

3. The stems -azepam and -azolam indicate that the

   drug is a _____.
   A. H_2 receptor antagonist
   B. Calcium channel blocker
   C. Corticosteroid
   D. Nonsteroidal anti-inflammatory drug (NSAID)
   E. Benzodiazepine

4. Select the **false** statement regarding synthetic and

   naturally derived drugs. _____
   A. A naturally derived drug may be a chemical modification of a synthetic drug.
   B. A synthetic drug may be manufactured entirely from chemical ingredients unrelated to a natural drug.
   C. Plants have been collected, cultivated, and harvested for their healing properties and used in the treatment of illness.
   D. Natural drugs may be derived from plants, animals, or minerals.

5. Select the **true** statement. _____
   A. The official name of a drug is the brand name.
   B. The proprietary name, or brand name, is assigned by the regulatory authority responsible for licensing the drug.
   C. Factors considered when selecting a suitable proprietary name are (1) whether an existing drug has a look-alike or sound-alike name and (2) whether the generic name can be easily associated with the name of an active ingredient in the new drug.
   D. The chemical name is the same as the generic name of the drug.

6. All of the statements about generic drugs are true

   except _____.
   A. a generic drug contains the same active ingredient as the original manufacturer's drug.
   B. a generic drug and its brand name equivalent have the same strength of the active ingredient and the same dosage form.
   C. generic drugs are more expensive than brand name drugs.
   D. a generic drug may contain different inactive ingredients than the brand name product.

7. Which of the following is true?
   A. Suspensions can be delivered orally, topically, or rectally.
   B. ODT tablets dissolve more slowly than sublingual tablets.
   C. Capsules are solid dosage forms that contain the active ingredient only.
   D. Delayed-action tablets are destroyed mostly in the stomach.

8. All of the following statements about the preparation and administration of parenterally administered

   drugs are true *except* _____.
   A. aseptic technique must be used when preparing drugs for parenteral administration.
   B. high doses of drugs administered intravenously (injected into a vein) must be injected rapidly to avoid destruction of red blood cells (hemolysis).
   C. drugs formulated for intramuscular administration (injected into a muscle) may produce a rapid onset or a slow onset of action.
   D. parenteral formulations may be administered intravenously, intramuscularly, or subcutaneously.

9. Select the drug formulation that has a slow onset of action and prolonged effects. _____
    A. Inhalation (e.g., metered-dose inhaler)
    B. Sublingual tablet (e.g., nitroglycerin)
    C. Intramuscular depot injection (e.g., prolixin decanoate)
    D. All of the above

10. Medications can be formulated for injection into the:
    A. Vein
    B. Muscle
    C. Cerebrospinal fluid
    D. Joint
    E. All of the above

MATCHING

Match the US legislation with its intended effect.

A. Durham-Humphrey amendment
B. Kefauver-Harris amendment
C. Drug Price Competition and Patent Term Restoration Act (1984)
D. Pure Food and Drug Act (1906)
E. National Association of Provincial Regulatory Authority Schedule II
F. Controlled Substance Act (1970)
G. Combat Methamphetamine Epidemic Act of 2005

1. The _____ requires that all drugs be safe and effective before they are made available to the public.

2. The _____ is the first significant legislation passed to protect the public from harmful and ineffective drugs.

3. The _____ encouraged the creation of generic drugs.

4. The _____ established the distinction between legend drugs and over-the-counter drugs.

5. The _____ was passed in order to regulate OTC sales of ephedrine, pseudoephedrine, and phenylpropanolamine.

6. The _____ regulates drugs that have a history of abuse

7. Behind-the-counter drugs in Canada are classified as _____, allowing patients to receive the drug without a prescription but with the security of a pharmacist's intervention

TRUE OR FALSE

1. _____ Egypt, Mesopotamia, India, and China have contributed to our body of knowledge of medicinals.

2. _____ A synthetic drug may be a chemical modification of a natural drug or manufactured entirely from chemical ingredients.

3. _____ The Drug Enforcement Agency regulates the new drug and investigational new drug process in the United States.

4. _____ The Health Products and Food Branch of Health Canada regulates the use of therapeutic drugs in Canada.

5. _____ The new drug application process includes preclinical research; clinical studies; phase 1, 2, and 3 trials; and postmarket safety studies.

6. _____ If a drug product contains multiple active ingredients, all official drug names must be listed on the medication label.

7. _____ In the United States, patent holders for new drugs are given up to 20 years' exclusive rights to manufacture and distribute the drugs.

8. _____ Generic drugs are often a cheaper option and must contain the same active *and* inactive ingredients as their brand name counterparts.

9. _____ A topically administered drug can produce a local effect only.

10. _____ Parenteral drugs with rapid onset of action are typically prepared in water-soluble solutions, and slow-onset, prolonged-duration-of-action formulations are suspended in oil or other nonaqueous vehicles (solvents).

CRITICAL THINKING

1. Why is it crucial for pharmacy technicians to practice aseptic technique when preparing drugs for parenteral administration?

_____

_____

_____

_____

_____

RESEARCH ACTIVITY

1. Conduct an Internet search of risk management plans to answer the following question: In Europe, manufacturers of new drugs must submit a risk management plan (EU-RMP) with their application for licensing. How might this practice help protect public health?

_____

_____

_____

_____

_____

CASE STUDY

A 6-year-old child comes into the hospital with severe pain. The physician on duty chooses to prescribe fentanyl to reduce the pain.

1. Research the different available drug products for fentanyl. What are the advantages and disadvantages of each?

_____

_____

_____

_____

_____

2. Which one(s) might be the best option for this patient?

_____

_____

_____

_____

3. As you noticed from your research, fentanyl is unavailable as a conventional tablet. Why do you think this is so?

_____

_____

_____

_____

2 Principles of Pharmacology

TERMS AND DEFINITIONS

Match each term with the correct definition below.

A. Absorption
B. Biotransformation
C. Distribution
D. Duration of action
E. Diffusion
F. Electrolytes
G. Enzyme
H. First-pass effect
I. Half-life
J. Hydrophilic
K. Hydrophobic
L. Ionization
M. Lipid
N. Lipophilic
O. Metabolism
P. Metabolite
Q. Peak effect
R. Pharmacokinetics
S. Prodrug

1. Osmosis is an example of the process of _____, which is the passive movement of molecules across cell membranes from an area of high drug concentration to an area of lower drug concentration.

2. The cytochrome P-450 system consists of _____ (s) capable of increasing the metabolism of drugs in the liver.

3. A product of metabolism, a _____ may be an inactivated drug or active drug with equal or greater activity than the parent drug.

4. The length of time it takes for the plasma concentration of an administered drug to be reduced by half is known as the

_____.

5. _____ is the chemical process involving the release of a proton (H^+). Ionized drug molecules may have a positive or negative charge.

6. Lipid-loving substances (_____) are _____ (water hating).

7. Small charged molecules involved with homeostasis are

_____.

8. A _____ is a drug that is administered in an inactive form and metabolized in the body to an active form.

9. _____ drugs are water loving.

10. During the pharmacokinetic phase of _____, the drug

undergoes _____, a process whereby the drug is converted to a more active, equally active, or inactive metabolite.

11. The first pharmacokinetic phase is _____, the process involving the movement of drug molecules from the site of administration into the circulatory system.

12. The _____ is the process whereby the liver metabolizes nearly all of a drug before it passes into the general circulation.

13. The maximum effect produced by a drug is known as the _____ and is achieved once the drug has reached its maximum concentration in the body.

14. _____ is the science dealing with the dynamic process a drug undergoes to produce its therapeutic effect.

15. A(n) _____ is a fatlike substance.

16. The process of movement of a drug from the circulatory system across barrier membranes to the site of drug action is called _____.

17. _____ is the time between the onset and discontinuation of drug action.

MULTIPLE CHOICE

1. Which of the following may be substituted for the brand name drug when authorized (i.e., follows product substitution laws)? _____
   A. Pharmaceutical alternative drug
   B. Pharmaceutical equivalent drug
   C. Bioequivalent drug
   D. Therapeutic alternative drug

2. Which of the following is *not* a pharmacokinetic phase? _____
   A. Disintegration
   B. Absorption
   C. Distribution
   D. Metabolism
   E. Elimination

3. The time it takes a drug to reach the concentration necessary to produce a therapeutic effect is the _____.
   A. site of action
   B. duration of action
   C. onset of action
   D. mechanism of action

4. The rate of absorption depends on the _____.
   A. lipid solubility
   B. extent of ionization
   C. surface area
   D. all of the above
   E. none of the above

5. Which drug is most likely to cross the blood-brain barrier? _____
   A. A lipid-soluble drug
   B. A drug that easily ionizable
   C. A hydrophilic drug
   D. A nonionized drug
   E. A and D

6. What factor would increase the bioavailability of a drug? _____
   A. Decreased drug absorption
   B. Increased first-pass effect
   C. Increased distribution of the drug
   D. Taking the drug orally rather than intravenously

7. Active drug transport _____.
   A. requires no energy
   B. can move a drug from a low to high concentration area
   C. is required to transport lipid-soluble drugs across the cell membrane
   D. is the method by which most drugs distribute throughout the body

8. The main organ for metabolism is the _____.
   A. kidney
   B. liver
   C. heart
   D. stomach

9. Metabolism of a drug can result in
   _____.
   A. converting a prodrug to its active form
   B. converting an active drug to an inactive metabolite
   C. converting an active drug to a more active metabolite
   D. all of the above
   E. none of the above

10. Premature infants are especially sensitive to drugs because of all of the following *except*
    _____.
    A. their kidneys are not well developed
    B. their drug-metabolizing capacity is limited
    C. their capacity for protein binding of drugs is excessive
    D. their lungs are not well developed

MATCHING

A. bioequivalent drug
B. pharmaceutical alternative
C. pharmaceutical equivalent
D. therapeutic alternative

1. A _____ contains the same active ingredient as the brand name drug; however, the strength and dosage form may be different.

2. A _____ shows no statistical differences in the rate and extent of absorption when it is administered in the same strength, dosage form, and route of administration as the brand name product.

3. A _____ contains an identical amount of active ingredient as the brand name drug but may have different inactive ingredients or be manufactured in a different dosage form.

4. A _____ contains different active ingredient(s) than the brand name drug yet produces the same desired therapeutic outcome.

MATCHING

A. Metabolism
B. Elimination
C. Hydrophilic
D. Lipophilic

1. _____ Process of biotransformation taking place in the liver

2. _____ Water loving

3. _____ Process of drug removal from the body

4. _____ Lipid loving

TRUE OR FALSE

1. _____ When taken orally, drugs must undergo disintegration and dissolution before absorption can take place.

2. _____ A synthetic drug may be a chemical modification of a natural drug or manufactured entirely from chemical ingredients.

3. _____ The first-pass effect describes why some drugs, if taken orally, would be inactivated before exerting an effect.

4. _____ Protein-bound drugs pass easily through capillary walls.

5. _____ Factors influencing metabolism are kidney function, disease, patient age, drug interactions, genetics, nutrition, and patient gender.

6. _____ When drugs are located in the basic solutions of the small intestine, it is the weakly acidic drugs that are absorbed more readily in comparison to weakly basic drugs.

7. _____ Drugs are absorbed across cell membranes via active and passive transport mechanisms.

CRITICAL THINKING

1. Compare and contrast pharmaceutical alternatives, pharmaceutical equivalents, bioequivalent drugs, and therapeutic alternatives. Relate your discussion to generic substitution.

_____

_____

_____

_____

_____

RESEARCH ACTIVITY

1. We typically think of drug interactions as bad. Conduct an Internet search of drug interactions to find examples of drugs that are administered concurrently for the beneficial effects of their interaction.

_____

_____

_____

_____

_____

2. How can pharmacy technicians help reduce harmful drug interactions?

_____

_____

_____

_____

_____

A new patient at the pharmacy was prescribed clopidogrel to prevent a stroke. Clopidogrel is a substrate of the CYP450 2C19 enzyme and becomes inactive when metabolized.

1. Identify the changes in peak effect and duration of action if the patient was also taking amiodarone.

_____

_____

_____

_____

_____

2. Identify the changes in peak effect and duration of action if the patient was also taking omeprazole.

_____

_____

_____

_____

_____

3. Identify the changes in peak effect and duration of action if the patient was also taking phenobarbital, a barbiturate.

_____

_____

_____

_____

_____

4. Clopidogrel is a prodrug. What does "prodrug" mean?

_____

_____

_____

_____

_____

3 Pharmacodynamics

TERMS AND DEFINITIONS

Match each term with the correct definition below.

A. Affinity
B. Agonist
C. Antagonist
D. Efficacy
E. Idiosyncratic reaction
F. Inverse agonist
G. Mechanism of action
H. Noncompetitive antagonist
I. Partial agonist
J. Pharmacodynamics
K. Pharmacotherapeutics
L. Potency
M. Receptor site
N. Therapeutic index

1. _____ is the study of drugs and their actions on a living organism.

2. An unexpected drug reaction is known as a(n) _____.

3. The use of drugs in the treatment of disease, _____, is the study of factors that influence the patient response to drugs.

4. The _____ is a ratio of the effective dose to the lethal dose.

5. _____ is the measure of a drug's effectiveness.

6. _____ is defined as the effective dose concentration.

7. _____ is defined as the attraction that the receptor site has for the drug.

8. The manner in which a drug produces its effect is the _____.

9. The drug that can turn "off" an activated receptor and turn "on" a receptor not currently active is known as a(n) _____.

10. A(n) _____ is a drug that binds to its receptor site and stimulates a cellular response.

11. A drug that binds to an alternative receptor site that prevents binding of an agonist is a(n) _____.

12. A binding drug that does not produce action is known as a(n) _____.

13. A(n) _____ behaves as an agonist under some conditions and acts as an antagonist under other conditions.

14. The location of drug-cell binding is known as the _____.

1. Select the statement about drug-receptor binding that

   is **false**. _____
   A. The more similar a drug is to the shape of a receptor site, the greater is the affinity the receptor site has for the drug.
   B. Drug-receptor binding may enhance or inhibit normal biological processes.
   C. An agonist is a drug that binds to its receptor site and stimulates a cellular response.
   D. Antagonist binding turns off a receptor that was activated.
   E. Drug-receptor binding is like a "lock and key."

2. Individual variation in pharmacokinetic and pharmacological responses may be caused by all of

   the following *except* the patient's _____.
   A. weight and gender
   B. emotional state
   C. age
   D. disease state
   E. hair color

3. Patients who have been diagnosed with

   _____ tend to experience more severe adverse drug reactions.
   A. Kidney disease
   B. Liver disease
   C. Lung disease
   D. All of the above

4. Which drug is most potent? _____

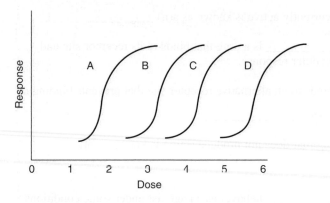

   A. Drug A
   B. Drug B
   C. Drug C
   D. Drug D

5. The basic requirement of a receptor is

   _____.
   A. recognition of molecules to bind and produce an effect in the cell
   B. that it fit only one drug
   C. that it is the place to deposit your genes
   D. none of the above

6. An elderly patient is likely to experience adverse drug reactions more frequently than an adolescent patient. Which factor primarily accounts for this?

   _____
   A. Drug clearance is more rapid in adolescents.
   B. Elderly patients are more likely to be taking multiple drugs than adolescent patients; therefore, drug elimination is slower in elderly patients.
   C. Adolescent patients have increased blood flow to the gastrointestinal tract.
   D. Higher doses are given to geriatric patients.

7. Which statement about drug dependence is **false**?

   _____
   A. Drug dependence is an adverse reaction that is associated with antibiotics.
   B. When dependence develops, a patient must take increasing doses of a drug to get the desired effect.
   C. When dependence has developed, a patient must continue to take a drug to prevent withdrawal symptoms.
   D. All drugs can produce dependence.

8. A drug that turns "off" a receptor that is normally activated is considered a(n):
   A. Competitive antagonist
   B. Inverse agonist
   C. Partial agonist
   D. None of the above

9. Mrs. Smith is picking up a new prescription for citalopram to treat depression. She thinks that "there's no way a small little pill is ever going to make me happy again." Based on this information, what factor is likely to affect her adherence to this medication?
   A. Dose schedule misunderstanding
   B. Ability to afford drug therapy
   C. Adverse drug reaction
   D. Perceived benefits of therapy

10. A pharmacy should report suspected adverse drug

   reactions to the _____.
   A. Drug Enforcement Agency (DEA)
   B. Food and Drug Administration (FDA)
   C. Centers for Disease Control and Prevention (CDC)
   D. board of pharmacy

MATCHING

A. teratogen
B. carcinogen
C. hepatotoxic drug
D. nephrotoxic drug

1. A _____ is able to produce a serious adverse reaction in the liver.

2. A _____ is able to produce a serious reaction in the kidney.

3. A _____ is able to produce harm to a developing fetus.

4. A _____ is able to stimulate the growth of cancers.

MATCHING

A. Ceiling effect
B. Potency
C. LD_{50}
D. Desensitization
E. ED_{50}

1. _____ Lethal dose for 50% of the population

2. _____ Maximum possible effect that could be produced

3. _____ Effective dose for 50% of the population

4. _____ Effective dose concentration

5. _____ Decreased drug response over time because of repeated exposure

TRUE OR FALSE

1. _____ Drugs that are administered in very low doses yet produce a maximum effect have high efficacy.

2. _____ A steep dose-response curve indicates that a large change in a drug dose is required to produce a big change in the drug response.

3. _____ Safe drugs have a wide margin between the lethal dose and the effective dose.

4. _____ Age, gender, disease, pregnancy, weight, and genetics are patient-related factors that influence the drug response.

5. _____ The placebo effect demonstrates that only biological factors are responsible for the patient response to drugs.

6. _____ Extended-release medications decrease patient adherence.

7. _____ Patients may develop tolerance to the side effects of a drug without developing tolerance to its therapeutic effects.

13

CRITICAL THINKING

1. Draw a dose-response curve. (Label the maximum therapeutic drug level and the ceiling effect.)

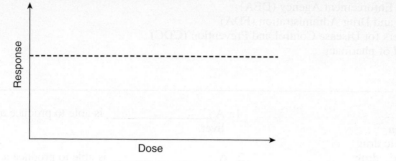

2. Write a short paragraph describing the relationship between the receptor site, agonists, and antagonists.

_____

_____

_____

_____

_____

RESEARCH ACTIVITY

1. What can pharmacy technicians do to reduce the patient's risk for adverse drug reactions, within the scope of practice for technicians?

_____

_____

_____

_____

2. What can pharmacy technicians do to increase patient adherence?

_____

_____

_____

_____

_____

CASE STUDY

An elderly patient comes into the pharmacy. When picking up his Benicar HCT to help lower his blood pressure, you notice that he should have been out of the medication 2 weeks ago. You ask him how his therapy has been going, and he responds by saying, "Not well. I've been keeping track of my blood pressure, and it's still high!"

1. Describe at least three potential reasons why this medication may not be working as intended for this patient.

_____

_____

_____

_____

_____

2. Describe what you, along with the pharmacist's help, could do to resolve any potential adherence problems with the patient.

_____

_____

_____

_____

_____

A few months later, the patient comes back to the pharmacy. According to his refill dates, you notice that his adherence to Benicar HCT has improved dramatically. You check his blood pressure journal and see that his most recent reading was 92/58, a level that is lower than desired. Upon further questioning, you also find out that he has liver disease. After consulting with the pharmacist, you understand that the current dose of Benicar HCT is too high.

3. Identify at least three physiological factors that could explain why the patient's dose of Benicar is changing his blood pressure levels so drastically.

_____

_____

_____

_____

_____

4. Benicar HCT has a relatively wide therapeutic index, so the patient was not harmed by the high dose. Explain the importance of proper adherence for lithium, warfarin, and other drugs that have narrow therapeutic indexes.

_____

_____

_____

_____

_____

4 Drug Interactions and Medication Errors

TERMS AND DEFINITIONS

Match each term with the correct definition below.

A. Additive effect
B. Antagonism
C. Drug-disease contraindication
D. Drug-drug interaction
E. Drug-food interaction
F. Medication error
G. Potentiation
H. Synergistic effects
I. Therapeutic duplication

1. An error made in the process of prescribing, preparing, dispensing, or administering drug therapy is called a _____.

2. An altered drug response that occurs when a drug is administered with certain foods is called _____.

3. Interactions between two drugs may produce _____ that are greater than would be produced if either drug were administered alone.

4. _____ is the administration of two drugs that produce similar therapeutic effects and side effects.

5. _____ is a reaction that occurs when two or more drugs are administered at the same time.

6. When administration of the drug may worsen the patient's medical condition, a(n) _____ exists.

7. An increased drug effect, or _____, is produced when a second similar drug is added to therapy and the effects produced are greater than the effects produced by either drug alone.

8. _____ is a process by which one drug or food, acting at a separate site or via a different mechanism of action, increases the effect of another drug, yet produces no effect when administered alone.

9. A drug-drug interaction or drug-food interaction that decreases or blocks the effects of another drug is called _____.

1. A drug interaction that can increase the risk for

   pregnancy may occur when _____
   is(are) taken with oral contraceptives.
   A. birth control pills
   B. amoxicillin
   C. aspirin
   D. antihistamines
   E. ibuprofen

2. Which of the following fruits is implicated in

   food-drug interactions? _____
   A. Apple
   B. Pear
   C. Grapefruit
   D. Plum
   E. Grape

3. Which vitamin may be administered as an antidote

   for the drug warfarin? _____
   A. Vitamin A
   B. Vitamin B
   C. Vitamin C
   D. Vitamin D
   E. Vitamin K

4. Which way of writing the milligram (mg) strength
   of a drug can reduce medication errors?

   _____
   A. 1.0 mg
   B. 1 mg
   C. 1.00 mg
   D. 01 mg

5. Which is *not* a characteristic of an "aseptic attitude"
   when preparing parenteral medications?

   _____
   A. Handwashing
   B. Hood cleaning
   C. Dose calculating
   D. Proper technique
   E. Eating in the clean room

6. Pharmacy technicians may reduce medication errors

   by all of the following *except* _____.
   A. always checking the original prescription against
      the prescription label and the NDC number (DIN
      number in Canada) on the stock bottle
   B. asking patients to spell sound-alike drugs when
      they call to request refills
   C. guessing what the medication might be when the
      handwriting on the prescription is difficult to read
   D. always placing a zero in front of the decimal
      point when calculating doses that are less than
      1 mL or 1 mg.
   E. writing legibly

7. Medication errors can happen at all the following

   times *except* when _____.
   A. Dispensing medication
   B. Administering medication
   C. Interpreting a written prescription
   D. Writing a medication order
   E. All of the above

8. Which statement about drug interactions is **false**?

   _____
   A. Drug interactions may be caused by induction or
      inhibition of metabolic enzymes.
   B. Interactions cannot be avoided by maintaining an
      up-to-date history of the patients' chronic and
      acute medical conditions.
   C. Interactions that involve competition for a
      common transport system in the kidney can
      affect the elimination of some drugs.
   D. Pharmacists and pharmacy technicians should
      screen all prescriptions for potential drug
      interactions before dispensing a medication.

9. When warfarin and _____ are
   administered together, excessive bleeding occurs.
   A. acetaminophen
   B. codeine
   C. penicillin
   D. aspirin

10. Which abbreviation can be found on the Joint

    Commission "Do Not Use" list? _____
    A. QD
    B. BID
    C. TID
    D. QID

MATCHING

A. "Chicken scratch"
B. "Sound-alike, look-alike" drug
   names
C. (ʒi)
D. NKDA
E. (ʒ)

1. _____ One dram

2. _____ Poor handwriting

3. _____ Ounce

4. _____ Zyprexa and Celexa

5. _____ No known drug allergies

MATCHING

A. Bagging error
B. Miscommunication
C. Improper medication preparation
D. Improper labeling
E. Product selection error

1. Incorrect directions on the bottle

2. Placing Jeni Smith's prescription together with Jenny Smith's prescription

3. Dispensing Prozac when the prescription asked for Prilosec

4. Mixing a sterile compound without washing your hands first

5. Interpreting a hastily made voicemail incorrectly

TRUE OR FALSE

1. _____ The pharmacy should collect information about a patient's use of over-the-counter drugs and enter it into the patient profile.

2. _____ NKDA is an abbreviation commonly used in pharmacies that means the patient does not have drug allergies.

3. _____ Pharmacy technicians unfamiliar with apothecary symbols may confuse the symbols for ounce and dram.

4. _____ The more drugs that are administered to a patient, the less likely it is that interactions will occur.

5. _____ Coadministration of drugs and foods can increase absorption, distribution, metabolism, or elimination.

6. _____ The process by which a drug, or a food, increases the effects of another drug, yet does not produce any effects when administered alone, is called antagonism.

7. _____ Intravenous solutions of acids and bases are incompatible, and when the solutions are combined, solid particles (precipitates) form.

8. _____ Studies indicate that between 7% and 22% of adverse drug reactions are caused by drug-drug interactions.

9. _____ Medication errors can be made by both health care professionals and patients.

10. _____ Medication errors associated with prescribers are often a result of carelessness.

CRITICAL THINKING

1. It is recommended that pharmacy technicians develop a routine to avoid medication errors associated with distractions. Write a routine for yourself that you believe will help you avoid making medication errors in the pharmacy.

_____

_____

_____

_____

2. Complete the missing information in the chart below, using your knowledge of dangerous abbreviations.

Abbreviation	Interpretation	Alternate interpretation
QD		
		Morphine sulfate
	Intravenous	
AU, AS, AD		
	Half-strength	
		Discontinue

RESEARCH ACTIVITY

1. Conduct an Internet search on medication errors. What is the scope of the problem in the United States and Canada? What are the costs to patients, the health care system, and society?

_____

_____

_____

_____

CASE STUDY

You work in a busy retail pharmacy located inside a grocery store, and the pharmacy manager has noticed a recent increase in the number of medication errors that are being made. Though these errors have been resolved before reaching the patient, the manager has decided to hold a team meeting to discuss error-prevention strategies.

1. Given the pharmacy location, what are at least three potential sources of distraction at this pharmacy? What can be done to reduce or eliminate those distractions?

_____

_____

_____

_____

2. You have personally noticed that a number of patients have mistakenly been given someone else's prescriptions. Describe two ways in which these errors occur and strategies to prevent each of them.

_____

_____

_____

_____

_____

A few months later, you apply for and accept a job inside a hospital pharmacy. You have little experience in this area of pharmacy, and you are nervous about making mistakes.

3. Compare the responsibilities of a retail pharmacy technician to a hospital pharmacy technician. What are the common sources of error in each setting?

_____

_____

_____

_____

4. What are the potential sources of distraction at this pharmacy? What can be done to reduce them in your workflow?

_____

_____

_____

_____

_____

21

5 Treatment of Anxiety

TERMS AND DEFINITIONS

Match each term with the correct definition below.

A. Anxiety
B. Anxiolytic
C. Drug dependence
D. Generalized anxiety disorder
E. Obsessive-compulsive disorder
F. Panic disorder
G. Phobia
H. Posttraumatic stress disorder
I. Tolerance

1. An irrational fear of things or situations, a(n) _____ produces symptoms of intense anxiety.

2. _____ is a condition associated with an inability to control or stop repeated unwanted thoughts or behaviors.

3. A stress disorder that develops in persons who have participated in, witnessed, or been a victim of a terrifying event is called a

   _____.

4. When a person must take increasing doses of a drug to achieve the same effects as were achieved at previously lower doses, he or she has

   developed _____.

5. _____ is a condition that is associated with excessive worrying and tension that is experienced daily for more than 6 months.

6. Repeated episodes of a sudden onset of feelings of terror are associated

   with _____.

7. _____ is a condition associated with tension, apprehension, fear, or panic.

8. When a person taking a drug must continue to take the drug to avoid the onset of physical and/or psychological withdrawal symptoms, he or she

   has developed _____.

9. A(n) _____ is a drug used to treat anxiety.

MULTIPLE CHOICE

1. Anxiety disorders are *not* linked to

   _____ factors.
   A. environmental
   B. societal
   C. biological
   D. developmental
   E. socioeconomic

2. The following statements are true about benzodiazepines *except*:
   A. Abrupt discontinuation of those with short half-lives precipitates withdrawal symptoms quickly.
   B. Abrupt discontinuation of those with long half-lives leads to delayed withdrawal symptoms.
   C. Most benzodiazepines are C-IV, although some are C-III.
   D. Benzodiazepines are sometimes used in surgeries because they can cause the patient to "forget" about the procedure and have less anxiety about future operations.

3. Which of the following is *not* an accepted medical

   treatment for anxiety? _____
   A. Administration of anxiolytics
   B. Psychotherapy
   C. Cognitive-behavioral therapy
   D. Self-administration of alcohol

4. Select the **false** statement. _____
   A. Benzodiazepines may produce tolerance and dependence.
   B. Benzodiazepines may be long acting, intermediate acting, or short acting.
   C. Benzodiazepines may induce amnesia.
   D. Benzodiazepines close chloride ion (Cl$^-$) channels.
   E. Benzodiazepines bind to receptor sites on the GABA$_A$ complex.

5. All of the following medications may be prescribed

   for anxiety *except* _____.
   A. selective serotonin reuptake inhibitors
   B. tricyclic antidepressants
   C. benzodiazepines
   D. opioids

6. Common physiological symptoms of anxiety include

   _____.
   A. heart palpitations
   B. nausea
   C. decreased heart rate
   D. A and B
   E. All of the above

7. A warning label that should be affixed to prescription vials for benzodiazepines is

   _____.
   A. AVOID PROLONGED EXPOSURE TO SUNLIGHT
   B. TAKE WITH LOTS OF WATER
   C. MAY BE HABIT FORMING
   D. AVOID ANTACIDS, DAIRY PRODUCTS, AND FE^{2+} PRODUCTS

8. Aside from anxiety, benzodiazepines can also be

   used for _____.
   A. insomnia
   B. muscle relaxation
   C. seizure disorders
   D. All of the above

9. Which pair of drugs used to treat anxiety does *not* produce tolerance or dependence?

   _____
   A. lorazepam and buspirone
   B. buspirone and hydroxyzine HCl
   C. hydroxyzine HCl and diazepam
   D. diazepam and alprazolam

FILL IN THE BLANK: DRUG NAMES

1. What is the **brand name** for alprazolam? _____

2. What is the **generic name** for Effexor XR? _____

3. What is the **brand name** for clonazepam? _____

4. What is the **generic name** for Valium? _____

5. What is the **brand name** for lorazepam? _____

6. What is the **brand name** for escitalopram (United States)? _____

7. What is the **brand name** for buspirone? _____

8. What is the **generic name** for Cymbalta? _____

9. What is the **brand name** for paroxetine? _____

10. What is the **brand name** for hydroxyzine HCl? _____

11. What is the **generic name** for Prozac? _____

12. What is the **brand name** for sertraline? _____

MATCHING

Match each drug to its pharmacological classification.

A. Benzodiazepines
B. Antidepressants
C. Miscellaneous (antihistamine)
D. Azapirones
E. Beta-adrenergic antagonist

1. _____ Clomipramine

2. _____ BuSpar

3. _____ Hydroxyzine HCl

4. _____ Alprazolam

5. _____ Propranolol

TRUE OR FALSE

1. _____ Anxiety disorders are the leading form of mental health illness.

2. _____ Treating OCD with antidepressants requires a lower dose and a shorter course of treatment when compared to treating depression.

3. _____ A drug classified as a controlled substance IV does not pose a risk for tolerance and dependence.

4. _____ Symptoms of anxiety are associated with hyperactivity of the autonomic nervous system.

5. _____ Most benzodiazepines bind to $GABA_A$ receptors. This interaction increases the affinity of GABA to its GABA receptors, opening more chloride ion channels in the process.

6. _____ Benzodiazepines can produce an amnesia that causes the person receiving the drug to "forget," reducing anxiety associated with future medical procedures.

7. _____ Some symptoms of serotonin syndrome include sedation, constipation, and decreased blood pressure.

8. _____ Propranolol may be administered to reduce palpitations caused by stage fright.

CRITICAL THINKING

The following hard copies are brought to your pharmacy for filling. Identify the prescription error(s). (You already have the patient's full address on file.) There may be one error, more than one error, or no errors at all.

```
Micheal Vessalago, MD     Date _____
        1221 Madison #310
        Anytown, USA
Pt. Name _____ Lillie Neville _____
Address _____

℞   buspirone #60
        i BID


Refills __6__
    Vessalago
_____      _____
Substitution permitted    Dispense as written
```

1. Spot the error in the following prescription:
   A. RF limit exceeded
   B. Incorrect dosage form
   C. Incorrect directions
   D. No strength written
   E. Quantity missing

```
Kathy Principi, MD      Date _____
        1145 Broadway
        Anytown, USA
Pt. Name _____ Ellen Wilbur-Jones _____
Address _____

℞   lorazepam 1mg
        1 tablet BID


Refills __1__
    Principi
_____      _____
Substitution permitted    Dispense as written
```

2. Spot the error in the following prescription:
   A. Quantity missing
   B. Strength incorrect
   C. Strength missing
   D. Directions incorrect
   E. Dosage form incorrect

```
Kathy Principi, MD      Date _____
        1145 Broadway
        Anytown, USA
Pt. Name _____ Preston Scott _____
Address _____

℞   clonazepam 25mg    #30
        1 BID for panic


Refills _____
    Principi
_____      _____
Substitution permitted    Dispense as written
```

3. Spot the error in the following prescription:
   A. Quantity missing
   B. Strength missing
   C. Strength incorrect
   D. Directions incorrect
   E. Dosage form incorrect

4. List six pairs of anxiolytic drugs that have look-alike or sound-alike issues.

DRUG NAME	LOOK-ALIKE OR SOUND-ALIKE DRUG

RESEARCH ACTIVITY

1. Access the National Library of Medicine website (medlineplus.gov/anxiety.html) to identify and list nonpharmacological methods for reducing anxiety.

_____

_____

_____

_____

2. Benzodiazepines are scheduled Class IV medications. What are examples of medications in Classes I, II, III, and V? List a few drugs or drug classes in each category. What are the main differences among the five classes?

_____

_____

_____

_____

_____

CASE STUDY

A patient was recently diagnosed with generalized anxiety disorder; she began to take alprazolam 4 weeks ago. Her doctor instructed her to use either one-half or one tablet as needed. Over the last 2 weeks the patient has needed to use the whole tablet to relieve her anxiety symptoms. She says, "I really don't want to become addicted to these pills. I think I am going to stop taking them."

1. What is the difference between tolerance and dependence?

_____

_____

_____

_____

2. What are some withdrawal symptoms this patient could experience if she suddenly stopped taking her alprazolam?

_____

_____

_____

_____

3. List at least three other medications that the pharmacist could recommend to the patient's doctor to help treat anxiety disorder without producing tolerance and dependence.

_____

_____

_____

_____

The patient's doctor prescribes escitalopram, an SSRI, to help treat her generalized anxiety disorder.

4. How quickly should the patient expect this medication to work?

_____

_____

_____

_____

_____

6 Treatment of Depression

TERMS AND DEFINITIONS

Match each term with the correct definition below.

A. Adjunct
B. Bipolar disorder
C. Enuresis
D. Major depression
E. Monoamine oxidase
F. Serotonin syndrome

1. _____ is an enzyme that is responsible for degradation of certain neurotransmitters such as NE, 5-HT, and DA.

2. Bedwetting, or _____, is characterized by uncontrollable urination during sleep.

3. _____, a potentially life-threatening adverse drug reaction, is characterized by symptoms of confusion, agitation, tremors, and increased blood pressure.

4. A mental health illness associated with sudden swings in mood between depression and periods of insomnia, racing thoughts, and distractibility is _____.

5. _____ is a mental health illness associated with persistent feelings of sadness, emptiness, or hopelessness that persist for several weeks.

6. A drug is classified as _____ therapy when it is used to complement the effects of another drug.

MULTIPLE CHOICE

1. Clinical depression is caused by a _____.
   A. decrease in brain acetylcholine
   B. decrease in brain histamine
   C. decrease in brain serotonin, norepinephrine, and dopamine
   D. deficiency of certain neurotransmitters

2. Depression can have the following effects *except* _____.
   A. reduced self-esteem
   B. reduced concentration
   C. increased eating
   D. decreased sleeping
   E. All of the above are effects of depression

3. Monoamine oxidase inhibitors that are used to treat depression primarily interfere with which enzyme?
   A. MAO_A
   B. MAO_B
   C. MAO_C
   D. Both A and B

4. A blockade of cholinergic (muscarinic) receptors can lead to _____.
   A. dry mouth
   B. diarrhea
   C. increased focus
   D. weight gain

5. Symptoms of bipolar disorder are _____.
   A. racing thoughts
   B. distractibility
   C. increased goal-directed behavior
   D. insomnia
   E. all of the above

6. What foods and beverages should be avoided in patients taking MAOIs?
   A. Foods high in sodium
   B. Foods high in tyramine
   C. Foods low in sodium
   D. Foods low in tyramine

7. Which of the following medications may be prescribed for enuresis?
   A. Fluoxetine and olanzapine
   B. Phenelzine and trazodone
   C. Imipramine and nortriptyline
   D. Duloxetine and bupropion

8. What is the main mechanism of action of TCAs?
   A. 5-HT reuptake inhibitor
   B. NE reuptake inhibitor
   C. DA reuptake inhibitor
   D. A and B

9. Select the drug that is *not* used in the treatment of bipolar disorder. _____
   A. lithium
   B. paroxetine
   C. carbamazepine
   D. divalproex sodium
   E. lamotrigine

FILL IN THE BLANK: DRUG NAMES

1. What is the *generic name* for Tofranil? _____

2. What is the *brand name* for desipramine? _____

3. What is a *brand name* for doxepin? _____

4. What is a *brand name* for trimipramine? _____

5. What is a *brand name* for nortriptyline? _____

6. What is the *generic name* for Lexapro (United States)? _____

7. What is the *brand name* for citalopram? _____

8. What is the *generic name* for Prozac? _____

9. What is the *generic name* for Luvox? _____

10. What is the *brand name* for paroxetine? _____

11. What is the *generic name* for Zoloft? _____

12. What is the *brand name* for phenelzine? _____

13. What is the *generic name* for Parnate? _____

14. What is the *brand name* for bupropion? _____

15. What is the *brand name* for mirtazapine? _____

16. What is the *generic name* for Desyrel? _____

17. What is the *brand name* for venlafaxine? _____

Chapter **6** **Treatment of Depression**

18. What is a **brand name** for lithium carbonate? _____

19. What is a **brand name** for carbamazepine? _____

20. What is the **generic name** for Lamictal? _____

MATCHING

Patient education is an essential component of therapeutics. Select the **best** warning label to apply to the prescription vial given to patients taking the drugs listed. An answer can be used more than once or not at all.

A. MAY DISCOLOR URINE
B. SWALLOW WHOLE; DO NOT CRUSH OR CHEW
C. AVOID PREGNANCY
D. AVOID TYRAMINE-CONTAINING FOODS
E. TAKE WITH FOOD

1. _____ Nardil 15 mg

2. _____ Effexor XR 75 mg

3. _____ Wellbutrin 150 mg SR

4. _____ Lithobid 300 mg

5. _____ amitriptyline 10 mg

MATCHING

Match each drug to its pharmacological classification.

A. tricyclic antidepressant (TCA)
B. selective serotonin reuptake inhibitor (SSRI)
C. monoamine oxidase inhibitor (MAOI)
D. serotonin-noradrenaline reuptake inhibitor (SNRI)
E. mood stabilizer/anticonvulsant

1. _____ Prozac 20 mg

2. _____ phenelzine 15 mg

3. _____ venlafaxine XR 75 mg

4. _____ imipramine HCL 10 mg

5. _____ carbamazepine ER 100 mg

MATCHING

Match each drug to its pharmacological classification. An answer can be used more than once or not at all.

A. tricyclic antidepressant (TCA)
B. selective serotonin reuptake inhibitor (SSRI)
C. serotonin-noradrenaline reuptake inhibitor (SNRI)
D. noradrenaline-dopamine inhibitor (NA/DRI)
E. monoamine oxidase inhibitor (MAOI)
F. atypical antidepressant

1. _____ bupropion 150 mg SR

2. _____ desipramine 50 mg

3. _____ moclobemide 100 mg

4. _____ duloxetine DR 30 mg

5. _____ paroxetine 20 mg

6. _____ mirtazapine 15 mg

TRUE OR FALSE

1. _____ Tricyclic antidepressants (TCAs) can increase cravings for sweets.

2. _____ Prescriptions for large quantities of TCAs may be written for depressed patients who are believed to be suicidal.

3. _____ Lithium has a narrow therapeutic index.

4. _____ A hypertensive crisis is a fatal adverse reaction associated with TCAs.

5. _____ Prescriptions for MAOIs should be dispensed with a list of tyramine-containing foods and a list of drugs to avoid.

6. _____ Contents of Effexor XR capsules cannot be sprinkled onto food.

7. _____ The endings -tyline and -pramine are commonly used for tricyclic antidepressants.

8. _____ A common ending for SSRIs is -oxetine.

9. _____ According to the biogenic amine theory, clinical depression results from an increase in monoamine neurotransmitters in the brain.

CRITICAL THINKING

The following hard copies are brought to your pharmacy for filling. Identify the prescription error(s). (You already have the patient's full address on file.) There may be one error, more than one error, or no errors at all.

Micheal Vessalago, MD   Date _____
1221 Madison #310
Anytown, USA

Pt. Name _____ Fatou Njie _____
Address _____ 2306 Broadway E Sea, WA _____

Rx   imipramine 10 mg, i qd x 3d, ii qd x 3d,
      iii qd x 3d, iv qd thereafter

Refills ___5___

___Vessalago___
Substitution permitted   Dispense as written

---

1. Spot the error in the following prescription:

   _____

   A. Quantity missing
   B. Strength missing
   C. Strength incorrect
   D. Directions missing
   E. Dosage form incorrect

Kathy Principi, MD   Date _____
1145 Broadway
Anytown, USA

Pt. Name _____ Will Jones _____
Address _____

Rx   amitriptyline 50mg tab   #30
      1 tablet

Refills _____

___Principi___
Substitution permitted   Dispense as written

---

2. Spot the error in the following prescription:

   _____

   A. Quantity missing
   B. Directions incomplete
   C. Strength missing
   D. Strength incorrect
   E. Dosage form incorrect

```
Anh Dang Tu, MD          Date _____
             1145 Broadway
             Anytown, USA

Pt. Name _____ Phuong Nguyen _____
Address _____

Rx   Wellbutrin 150mg SR tab     #60
        i tab QID



Refills _____
        A. Tu
_____
Substitution permitted      Dispense as written
```

3. Spot the error in the following prescription:

   _____

   A. Quantity missing
   B. Strength missing
   C. Strength incorrect
   D. Directions incorrect
   E. Dosage form incorrect

```
Kathy Principi, MD        Date _____
             1145 Broadway
             Anytown, USA

Pt. Name _____ Preston Scott _____
Address _____

Rx   fluoxetine capsules
        1 g AM



Refills __2__
        Principi
_____
Substitution permitted      Dispense as written
```

4. Spot the error in the following prescription:

   _____

   A. Quantity missing
   B. Strength missing
   C. DEA number missing
   D. Directions incorrect
   E. Dosage form incorrect

5. Write a short paragraph comparing and contrasting the mechanisms of action of TCAs, SSRIs, and MAOIs.

_____

_____

_____

_____

_____

6. How many tablets are required to fill Crystal Boelle's prescription for amitriptyline?

   Amitriptyline 25 mg i QD × 3 days, ii QD × 3 days; iii QD × 3 days, iv QD thereafter.

   Dispense a 1-month supply, and please show your calculations.

_____

_____

_____

_____

_____

7. List six pairs of antidepressant drugs that have look-alike or sound-alike issues.

DRUG NAME	LOOK-ALIKE OR SOUND-ALIKE DRUG

RESEARCH ACTIVITY

1. Sheila Bogan calls to refill her antidepressant medication. She does not remember the name. Review her patient profile, and make a list of the drugs used to treat depression. Search the Internet to find pictures of the drugs, and then develop a list of questions you might ask to identify the drug she is requesting.

Last Name: Bogan	First Name: Sheila	Gender: F
Address: 1310 34th Ave. S #310	City: Anytown	DOB: 12-14-53
Allergies: NKA	Disc:	Phone: 725-2743
Insurance: PCS	Plan: 05	Group: 54873456
ID: 536234177	Copay: $10.00/$20.00	
Cardholder: Kargan	Melinda	Exp. date:

DATE	RX#	DRUG AND STRENGTH	SIG	QTY	MD	RF
10-2-07	72345	amitriptyline 50 mg	1 HS	60	Johnson, C	2
11-1-07	72345	amitriptyline 50 mg	1 HS	60	Johnson, C	1
12-2-07	81956	meperidine 100 mg	1 q6h PRN	20	Hohl DDS	0
12-2-07	84358	Anaprox DS	1 BID	30	Hohl DDS	1
1-2-08	85345	trazodone 50 mg	1 HS	30	Johnson, C	0
2-4-08	89278	Hycotuss	5–10 mL q6h	240	Johnson, C	3
2-4-08	96346	Paxil CR 25 mg	1 qd	30	Ng, A	2
3-12-08	102344	Darvocet N 100	1 q6h	25	Ng, A	1
3-12-08	102345	bupropion 150 mg SR	1 BID	60	Ng, A	1
4-4-08	102345	bupropion 150 mg SR	1 q12h	60	Johnson, C	2
5-4-08	103366	Effexor 75 mg XR	1 q12h	60	Johnson, C	1

Make a list of the antidepressant drugs listed in the profile.

Make a list of questions you might ask to identify the current drug she is requesting.

ANTIDEPRESSANT DRUG	DRUG IDENTIFICATION QUESTIONS
	1.
	2.
	3.

2. Lithium is a medication with many drug interactions. Research to find some examples and describe this interaction if possible. Lithium also interacts with sodium in the kidneys; research the reason behind this interaction. (Hint: Examine the Periodic Table of Elements.)

CASE STUDY

A patient comes to your pharmacy to drop off a prescription for amitriptyline. He says, "I'm not sure I want this filled. I haven't been feeling like myself for a few months. My doctor says I have depression, but starting medication for depression makes me feel like a failure. I should be able to deal with my feelings on my own."

1. Using your knowledge of the biogenic amine theory, describe the role neurotransmitters (norepinephrine, serotonin, and dopamine) have in depression

_____

_____

_____

_____

2. Describe the mechanism of action of amitriptyline.

_____

_____

_____

_____

Three months later, the patient returns to the pharmacy and says he has not been using his amitriptyline because he doesn't like the side effects. He is still feeling depressed and wants to know whether there is anything he can do to minimize side effects.

3. List common adverse effects associated with tricyclic antidepressants.

_____

_____

_____

_____

The pharmacist explains that all antidepressants are equally effective, and she recommends that the patient talk to his doctor about switching to an SSRI. The next week, the patient brings in a new prescription for sertraline.

4. No medication is without side effects. What adverse effects would the patient possibly experience with sertraline?

_____

_____

_____

_____

_____

5. Serotonin syndrome is a rare but serious side effect associated with SSRIs. Describe the symptoms of serotonin syndrome.

_____

_____

_____

_____

Treatment of Schizophrenia and Psychoses

TERMS AND DEFINITIONS

Match each term with the correct definition below.

A. Catatonia
B. Delusion
C. Extrapyramidal symptoms
D. Hallucination
E. Negative symptoms
F. Neuroleptic (antipsychotic)
G. Neuroleptic malignant syndrome
H. Positive symptoms
I. Postural hypotension
J. Pseudoparkinsonism
K. Psychosis
L. Schizophrenia
M. Tardive dyskinesia

1. A(n) _____ is a drug used to treat schizophrenia and psychoses.

2. Potentially fatal, _____ produces symptoms such as stupor, muscle rigidity, and high temperature.

3. Persons with schizophrenia may exhibit _____ such as hallucinations, delusions, or other unusual thoughts.

4. A(n) _____ is a mental state characterized by disorganized behavior and thought, delusions, hallucinations, and a loss of touch with reality.

5. _____ is a symptom of schizophrenia that is associated with unresponsiveness and immobility.

6. The administration of neuroleptics may cause _____, excessive muscle movement, and difficulty in walking.

7. The term for a sudden drop in blood pressure upon a change in posture is

_____.

8. The administration of neuroleptics may produce _____, an adverse reaction that mimics Parkinson's disease.

9. Persons with schizophrenia may have a(n) _____, which presents as irrational thoughts or false beliefs that do not change even when evidence is provided that beliefs are not valid.

10. The administration of neuroleptics may produce _____, an adverse reaction that causes involuntary thrusting of the tongue and changes in posture.

11. Persons with schizophrenia may exhibit _____, which present as a decreased ability to think, plan, or express emotion.

12. _____ is a type of psychosis characterized by delusions of thought, visual and/or auditory hallucinations, and speech disturbances.

13. Visions or voices that exist only in the mind and cannot be seen or heard

by others are called a(n) _____.

MULTIPLE CHOICE

1. Neuroleptic malignant syndrome is characterized by symptoms of _____.
   A. hypothermia
   B. liver failure
   C. muscle rigidity
   D. B and C

2. Treatment for schizophrenia that involves dopamine blockade can produce _____.
   A. delusions
   B. neurolepsy
   C. psychosis
   D. pseudoparkinsonism

3. Paul Bunyan was institutionalized for schizophrenia. He was administered fluphenazine HCl, 2.5 mg IM every 6 hours, initially but has been switched to fluphenazine decanoate in preparation for discharge.

   Fluphenazine decanoate _____.
   A. is a slow-release preparation that is administered every 3 weeks
   B. should be dispensed with an oral syringe
   C. must be diluted in water or juice before administration
   D. is administered sublingually

4. Side effects of aripiprazole include

   _____.
   A. insomnia
   B. increased risk of death in patients with dementia
   C. hyperglycemia
   D. All of the above

5. Patients receiving chlorpromazine oral concentrate, 100 mg/mL, should be given the following advice:

   _____
   A. MAY CAUSE DROWSINESS OR DIZZINESS
   B. AVOID ALCOHOL
   C. DILUTE WITH LIQUID BEFORE INGESTION
   D. AVOID PROLONGED EXPOSURE TO SUNLIGHT
   E. All of the above

6. Dopamine antagonism in the _____ leads to symptoms of pseudoparkinsonism.
   A. nigrostriatal tract
   B. mesolimbic system
   C. substantia nigra
   D. hypothalamus

7. Which of the following statements about typical antipsychotics is true?
   A. Typical antipsychotics are much more clinically effective than atypical antipsychotics.
   B. Newer atypical antipsychotics are associated with less risk for extrapyramidal side effects.
   C. Medium-potency antipsychotics are associated with sedative and anticholinergic effects.
   D. Atypical antipsychotics can only be given orally; they are prodrugs that must go through the first-pass effect in the liver to be effective.

8. Peripheral nervous system side effects of

   antipsychotics include _____.
   A. constipation
   B. sedation
   C. urinary retention
   D. A and C

9. Up to _____ of the people who are prescribed neuroleptics will experience adverse reactions.
   A. 20%
   B. 40%
   C. 60%
   D. 80%
   E. 100%

10. Clozapine use is restricted because this drug can

    produce a fatal drop in the _____.
    A. white blood cell level
    B. red blood cell level
    C. blood pressure
    D. pulse

FILL IN THE BLANK: DRUG NAMES

1. What is the *generic name* for Invega (United States)? _____

2. What is the *generic name* for Modecate (Canada)? _____

3. What is a *brand name* for olanzapine? _____

4. What is the *generic name* for Saphris? _____

5. What is the *generic name* for Abilify? _____

6. What is the *brand name* for lurasidone? _____

7. What is the *brand name* for fluphenazine? _____

8. What is a *brand name* for quetiapine? _____

9. What is the *generic name* for Clozaril (United States)? _____

10. What is the *generic name* for Fanapt? _____

11. What is the *generic name* for Loxitane (United States)? _____

MATCHING

Match each drug to its pharmacological classification.

A. phenothiazines
B. benzisoxazoles
C. thioxanthenes
D. dibenzothiazepines
E. thienobenzodiazepines

1. _____ Navane

2. _____ clozapine

3. _____ Seroquel

4. _____ fluphenazine

5. _____ Risperdal

TRUE OR FALSE

1. _____ Haloperidol and risperidone oral concentrates should not be mixed with coffee or tea.

2. _____ Patients, prescribers, and pharmacists must be enrolled in a registry to dispense clozapine.

3. _____ The dropper that comes packaged with oral concentrate may be interchanged with other droppers and dispensed with the medicine.

4. _____ The greater the affinity a neuroleptic drug has for dopamine (D_2) receptors, the less effective is the drug.

5. _____ Schizophrenia affects about 1% of the population worldwide. Symptoms typically begin in the early to mid-20s and may not develop until the early 30s.

6. _____ Although dopamine is the most relevant neurotransmitter in schizophrenia, others play a role, including serotonin, cholecystokinin, and glutamate.

7. _____ Atypical antipsychotics have a strong affinity for dopamine receptors and often produce Parkinson's disease–like symptoms.

CRITICAL THINKING

The following hard copies are brought to your pharmacy for filling. Identify the prescription error(s). (You already have the patient's full address on file.) There may be one error, more than one error, or no errors at all.

Micheal Vessalago, MD   Date _____
1221 Madison #310
Anytown, USA

Pt. Name _____ G.W. Bushe _____
Address _____

℞   Zyprexa   #30
    10mg daily

Refills __3__

_Vessalago_____   _____
Substitution permitted   Dispense as written

---

1. Spot the error in the following prescription:

_____

A. Quantity missing
B. Strength missing
C. Strength incorrect
D. Directions missing
E. Dosage form incorrect

Anh Dang Tu, MD   Date _____
1145 Broadway
Anytown, USA

Pt. Name _____ Lili Ng _____
Address _____

℞   Prolixin decanoate 25mg/ml
    0.5 ml IM BID
    10ml

Refills __1__

_A. Tu_____   _____
Substitution permitted   Dispense as written

---

2. Spot the error in the following prescription:

_____

A. Quantity missing
B. Strength missing
C. Strength incorrect
D. Directions incorrect
E. Dosage form incorrect

Kathy Principi, MD   Date _____
1145 Broadway
Anytown, USA

Pt. Name _____ Preston Scott _____
Address _____

℞   Risperdal 1mg
    i bid x 1d; ii bid 2d; iii bid

Refills _____

_Principi_____   _____
Substitution permitted   Dispense as written

---

3. Spot the error in the following prescription:

_____

A. Quantity missing
B. Strength missing
C. DEA number missing
D. Directions incorrect
E. Dosage form incorrect

4. List three pairs of examples of neuroleptic drugs that have sound-alike or look-alike issues.

DRUG NAME	LOOK-ALIKE OR SOUND-ALIKE DRUG

5. Susan Kraft has been prescribed haloperidol, 2.5 mg twice a day. The pharmacy stocks 0.5-mg tablets. How many tablets will she need to take per day? Please show your calculations.

_____

_____

_____

_____

6. Nick Harper has previously been taking chlorpromazine, 50 mg PO every 6 hours. He has recently been hospitalized, and his medication has been changed from an oral to an intramuscular preparation (50 mg IM every 6 hours). Chlorpromazine HCl for parenteral use is available as 25 mg/mL. How many milliliters will you need to draw up into each syringe and send to his nursing unit? Please show your calculations.

_____

_____

_____

_____

7. Patient Sandra Smith has been taking Abilify, 5 mg twice daily. You check your shelf and see that the only Abilify product in stock is the 2-mg tablet. The patient states that she has a pill splitter at home. How many 2-mg tablets should you give the patient to fill a 7-day supply? How many tablets should the patient take for each dose? Please show your calculations.

_____

_____

_____

_____

RESEARCH ACTIVITY

1. Sheila Bogan calls to refill her medication. She does not remember the name. Review her patient profile, and make a list of the neuroleptic medications. Search the Internet to find pictures of the drugs, and then develop a list of questions you might ask to identify the drug she is requesting.

Last Name: Bogan   First Name: Sheila   Gender: F

Address: 1310 34th Ave. S #310   City: Anytown   DOB: 12-14-53

Allergies: NKA   Disc: Phone: 725-2743

Insurance: PCS   Plan: 05   Group: 54873456

ID: 536234177   Copay: $10.00/$20.00

Cardholder: Kargan   Melinda   Exp. date:

DATE	RX#	DRUG AND STRENGTH	SIG	QTY	MD	RF
10-2-07	72345	fluphenazine 5 mg	1 q8h	90	Johnson, C	2
11-1-07	72345	fluphenazine 5 mg	1 q8h	90	Johnson, C	1
12-2-07	81956	meperidine 100 mg	1 q6h PRN	20	Hohl DDS	0
12-2-07	84358	Anaprox DS	1 BID	30	Hohl DDS	1
1-2-08	85345	fluphenazine 25 mg/mL	12.5 mg q3wk	5 mL	Johnson, C	0
1-21-08	85345	fluphenazine 25 mg/mL	12.5 mg q3wk	5 mL	Johnson, C	0
2-4-08	89278	Hycotuss	5–10 mL q6h	240 mL	Johnson, C	3
2-4-08	96346	Risperdal 2 mg	1 BID	60	Ng, A	2
3-3-08	96346	Risperdal 2 mg	1 BID	60	Ng, A	1
4-2-08	102345	Risperdal 3 mg	1 BID	60	Ng, A	1
5-1-08	103366	Zyprexa Zydis 5 mg	2 daily	60	Johnson, C	1

Make a list of neuroleptic drugs contained in the profile.

Make a list of questions you might ask to identify the current drug she is requesting.

NEUROLEPTIC DRUG	DRUG IDENTIFICATION QUESTIONS
	1.
	2.
	3.

41

CASE STUDY

John is a patient who has been coming to your pharmacy for many years. His facial expressions are flat, he doesn't show emotion, and he has a hard time interacting with pharmacy staff members. He will often talk to himself. A new technician comes to you, complains that John was rude to her, and asks you what is wrong with him. You explain that John has schizophrenia.

1. Distinguish the differences between negative and positive symptoms of schizophrenia. Give examples of each.

_____

_____

_____

_____

_____

2. You receive a new prescription from John's doctor and in the notes he has written, "To treat extrapyramidal symptoms." What are extrapyramidal symptoms? Include examples.

_____

_____

_____

_____

3. John also has diabetes. List two medications that would be poor choices to treat John's schizophrenia due to their risk of causing hyperglycemia.

_____

_____

John is upset that he cannot refill one of his atypical antipsychotics because he forgot to go to his doctor's office to have his blood drawn. You explain to him that you must have the appropriate lab values to report to a special registry before you can dispense this medication.

4. Which medication is John trying to refill today?

_____

5. What value is being monitored by this lab work, and why is it important?

_____

_____

_____

_____

8 Treatment of Alzheimer's, Huntington's, and Parkinson's Disease

TERMS AND DEFINITIONS

Match each term with the correct definition below.

A. Acetylcholinesterase
B. Alzheimer's disease
C. ApoE4 allele
D. Bradykinesia
E. Cognitive function
F. Dementia
G. Huntington's disease
H. Neurodegeneration
I. Neuroprotective
J. Parkinson's disease
K. Plaques
L. Pseudoparkinsonism
M. Tangles

1. _____ is the progressive destruction of neurons.

2. The ability to take in information via the senses, process the details, commit the information to memory, and recall it when necessary is a(n) _____.

3. The enzyme that degrades the neurotransmitter acetylcholine is called _____.

4. The defective form of apolipoprotein E that is associated with Alzheimer's disease is called the _____.

5. _____ are twisted fibers made up of tau that interfere with signal transmission.

6. A condition associated with memory loss is referred to as _____.

7. _____ is a drug-induced condition that resembles Parkinson's disease.

8. The term used to describe slowness in initiating and carrying out voluntary movements is _____.

9. _____ and _____ are progressive disorders of the nervous system that impair muscle movement.

10. _____ is a neurodegenerative disease that causes memory loss and behavioral changes.

11. _____ agents protect nerve cells from damage.

12. Substances composed of beta amyloid called _____ fill the spaces between neurons and interfere with the transmission of signals between neurons.

1. What is Parkinson's disease? _____
   A. A progressive and degenerative disease in newborns
   B. A drug-induced condition
   C. A disease resulting from a vitamin deficiency
   D. A progressive disorder of the nervous system

2. Entacapone and tolcapone are COMT inhibitors and boost the bioavailability of levodopa by

   _____.
   A. 10%
   B. 50%
   C. 0.5%
   D. 75%

3. Approximately _____ million people in the United States have Parkinson's disease.
   A. 5
   B. 10
   C. 2
   D. 1

4. Which of the following statements is **false**?
   A. Sustained-release formulations of carbidopa/levodopa decrease bioavailability of the drug by 30% when compared to immediate-release formulations.
   B. The efficacy of levodopa remains fairly constant throughout the progression of Parkinson's disease.
   C. COMT inhibitors are used as adjunctive therapy to increase levodopa bioavailability by as much as 50%.
   D. Side effects of carbidopa/levodopa therapy include hallucinations, nausea/vomiting, and hypotension.

5. All of the following can be used to treat Parkinson's

   disease *except* _____.
   A. Duodopa
   B. levodopa
   C. bromocriptine
   D. Miralax

6. Which adverse effect is *not* associated with

   anticholinergic drugs? _____
   A. Dry mouth
   B. Diarrhea
   C. Blurred vision
   D. Constipation
   E. Urinary retention

7. Huntington's disease differs from Parkinson's disease

   because _____.
   A. Huntington's disease is a progressive and degenerative disease of neurons
   B. Huntington's disease affects muscle movement, cognitive functions, and emotions
   C. Huntington's disease is primarily treated with drugs that decrease excessive dopaminergic activity
   D. Huntington's disease symptoms are caused by an imbalance between neurotransmitters (e.g., acetylcholine, dopamine, and GABA)

8. Parkinson's disease is treated with

   _____.
   A. pharmaceuticals
   B. exercise
   C. nutritional support
   D. all of the above

9. Huntington's disease is primarily treated with drugs

   that decrease excessive _____ activity.
   A. cholinergic
   B. acetylcholinesterase
   C. dopaminergic
   D. norepinephrine

10. Which of the following drugs is indicated for the treatment of Huntington's disease?

    _____
    A. Requip
    B. Xenazine
    C. Nitroman
    D. Haldol

FILL IN THE BLANK: DRUG NAMES

1. What is the **brand name** for amantadine? _____

2. What is the **brand name** for haloperidol? _____

3. What is the **generic name** for Stalevo (United States)? _____

4. What is a **brand name** for levodopa and carbidopa? _____

5. What is the *generic name* for Mirapex? _____

6. What is the *generic name* for Requip? _____

7. What is the *brand name* for levodopa and benserazide? _____

8. What is a *brand name* for benztropine? _____

9. What is the *generic name* for Lodosyn? _____

10. What is a *brand name* for tetrabenazine? _____

MATCHING

Match each drug to its pharmacological classification or brand or generic name.

A. anticholinergic
B. dopamine agonist
C. tolcapone
D. MAOB inhibitor
E. levodopa

1. _____ Azilect

2. _____ trihexyphenidyl

3. _____ Mirapex

4. _____ dopamine precursor

5. _____ COMT inhibitor

MATCHING

Patient education is an essential component of therapeutics. Select the **best** warning label to apply to the prescription vial given to patients taking the drugs listed.

A. AVOID FOODS HIGH IN TYRAMINE
B. SWALLOW WHOLE; DO NOT CRUSH
C. TAKE WITH FOOD
D. MAY DISCOLOR URINE

1. _____ Mirapex ER 0.75mg

2. _____ selegiline 5 mg

3. _____ galantamine 4 mg

4. _____ Tasmar 100 mg

TRUE OR FALSE

1. _____ Bradykinesia will speed up voluntary movements.

2. _____ Parkinson's disease is associated with other mental diseases, including depression and dementia.

3. _____ Cognitive functions are not involved in the ability to take information in via the senses, process the details, commit the information to memory, or recall the information when necessary.

4. _____ Huntington's disease causes immobility while Parkinson's disease causes excessive movements.

5. _____ Carbidopa and benserazide are only used to reduce degradation of levodopa before it reaches the brain.

CRITICAL THINKING

The following hard copies are brought to your pharmacy for filling. Identify the prescription error(s). (You already have the patient's full address on file.) There may be one error, more than one error, or no errors at all.

```
        Micheal Vessalago, MD      Date _____
              1221 Madison #310
              Anytown, USA

Pt. Name _____ Marge Simpson _____
Address _____
Rx    Parlodel 2.5mg
         1 tab q 12 h


Refills ___6___
_____Vessalago_____        _____
Substitution permitted       Dispense as written
```

1. Spot the error in the following prescription:

   _____

   A. Quantity missing
   B. Strength missing
   C. Strength incorrect
   D. Directions missing
   E. Dosage form incorrect

```
        Kathy Principi, MD      Date _____
              1145 Broadway
              Anytown, USA

Pt. Name _____ Homer Wollensky _____
Address _____
Rx    Levodopa/carbidopa  #90
         1 tab TID


Refills  PRN
_____Principi_____        _____
Substitution permitted       Dispense as written
```

2. Spot the error in the following prescription:

   _____

   A. Quantity missing
   B. Directions incomplete
   C. Strength missing
   D. Strength incorrect
   E. Dosage form incorrect

```
        Marc Cordova, MD      Date _____
              1145 Broadway
              Anytown, USA

Pt. Name _____ Bill Carey _____
Address _____
Rx    Benztropine 0.5mg tab q 12 hours




Refills _____
_____Cordova_____        _____
Substitution permitted       Dispense as written
```

3. Spot the error in the following prescription:

   _____

   A. Quantity missing
   B. Directions incomplete
   C. Strength missing
   D. Strength incorrect
   E. Dosage form incorrect

4. Draw a picture to show the changes that occur in neurotransmitter levels in Parkinson's disease. BE SURE TO LABEL THE DIAGRAMS.

WITHOUT PARKINSON'S DISEASE	WITH PARKINSON'S DISEASE

5. List two pairs of drug names that have look-alike or sound-alike issues with drugs used to treat Parkinson's disease or Huntington's disease.

DRUG NAME	LOOK-ALIKE OR SOUND-ALIKE DRUG

RESEARCH ACTIVITY

1. Clark Kent calls to renew his Parkinson's disease medication. He does not remember the name of the drug. Review his patient profile, and make a list of the drugs for Parkinson's disease. Search the Internet to find pictures of the drugs, and then develop a list of questions you might ask to identify the drug he is requesting.

Last Name: Kent   First Name: Clark   Gender: M

Address: 1310 34th Ave. S #310   City: Anytown   DOB: 12-14-51

Allergies: NKA   Disc: Phone: 725-2743

Insurance: PCS Plan: 05   Group: 54873456   ID: 536234177   Copay: $7.00/$10

DATE	RX#	DRUG AND STRENGTH	MD	RF
11-7-06	236742	Sinemet 10–100 mg #90	Jones MD	2
12-05-06	236742	Sinemet 10–100 mg #90	Jones MD	1
1-4-07	236755	Sinemet 25–100 mg #90	Jones MD	0
1-4-07	236756	Phenytoin 100 mg #90	Jones MD	2
2-3-07	321477	Sinemet 25–100 mg CR #120	Jones MD	4
2-3-07	236756	Phenytoin ER 100 mg #90	Jones MD	1
3-2-07	321477	Sinemet 25–100 mg CR #120	Jones MD	3
3-26-07	344580	Demerol 100 mg #18	Bean DDS	0
3-26-07	344581	Amoxil 500 mg #9	Bean DDS	1
4-5-07	384222	Tegretol XR 300 mg #60	Jones MD	0
4-5-07	384223	benztropine 0.5 mg #30	Jones MD	0
5-13-07	384883	amitriptyline 10 mg #30	Jones MD	2
5-22-07	385129	Keppra 500 mg #60	Jones MD	1
5-22-07	385130	selegiline 5 mg #30	Jones MD	1

Make a list of the antiparkinson medications listed in his profile. (Give the brand and generic names.)

Make a list of questions you might ask to identify the current drug he is requesting.

ANTIPARKINSON DRUG	DRUG IDENTIFICATION QUESTIONS
	1.
	2.
	3.

CASE STUDY

You are helping Susan at your pharmacy counter. Susan is a good customer of yours, and so is her mother, Mary. You tell Susan you have missed seeing Mary at the pharmacy lately. Susan explains that she has been taking care of Mary's medications because Mary has been getting more and more forgetful. "But that's all part of getting old, right?" Susan says.

1. List some characteristics that would be concerning for Alzheimer's disease compared with normal aging.

_____

_____

_____

_____

_____

2. List two risk factors for developing Alzheimer's disease and at least three comorbid conditions that may speed the progression of the disease.

_____

_____

_____

_____

_____

A few months later, Susan returns to the pharmacy after Mary has a visit with her physician. She tells you that Mary has been diagnosed with Alzheimer's disease. She gives you a prescription for donepezil.

3. Describe the mechanism of action of donepezil and the role acetylcholine plays in Alzheimer's disease.

_____

_____

_____

_____

_____

_____

4. List some side effects Mary may experience after starting donepezil.

_____

_____

_____

_____

Susan tells the pharmacist she has been feeling very overwhelmed by her mother's new diagnosis. She is worried that she will also develop Alzheimer's disease.

5. What are some nonpharmacological measures Susan can take to reduce her risk for Alzheimer's disease?

_____

_____

_____

_____

_____

9 Treatment of Seizure Disorders

TERMS AND DEFINITIONS

Match each term with the correct definition below.

A. Anoxia
B. Aura
C. Complex focal seizures
D. Convulsions
E. Eclampsia
F. Epilepsy
G. Febrile seizure
H. Generalized seizures
I. Gingival hyperplasia
J. Hirsutism
K. Myoclonic seizure
L. Absence seizure
M. Seizure threshold
N. Simple focal seizures
O. Status epilepticus

1. The term that refers to a person's susceptibility to seizures is

   _____.

2. _____ is defined as a recurrent seizure disorder characterized by a sudden excessive, disorderly discharge of cerebral neurons.

3. The term used to describe excessive growth of body hair (especially in women) is _____.

4. A _____ is associated with a sudden spike in body temperature.

5. _____ is a medical emergency brought on by repeated generalized seizures that can produce _____, a lack of oxygen to the brain.

6. _____ is/are characterized by a sudden contraction of muscles and is/are caused by seizures.

7. The term used to describe the condition in which gum tissue overgrows the teeth is _____.

8. A(n) _____ is an unusual sensation or auditory, visual, or olfactory hallucination that is experienced just before the onset of a seizure.

9. _____ is characterized by brief periods of unconsciousness and vacant stares.

10. _____ affect only one part of the brain and cause the person to experience unusual sensations or feelings.

11. _____ is/are a disorder that produces a blank stare, disorientation, repetitive actions, and memory loss.

12. _____ is a life-threatening condition that can develop in pregnant women.

13. _____ include tonic-clonic, myoclonic, and absence seizures.

14. A _____ is a seizure that is characterized by jerking muscle movements and is caused by contraction of the major muscle groups.

MULTIPLE CHOICE

1. The World Health Organization estimates that

   _____ people worldwide have epilepsy.
   A. 2.2 million
   B. 5 million
   C. 50 million
   D. 1 billion

2. Seizures may be caused by all of the following *except*

   _____.
   A. infection and high fevers
   B. anxiety and schizophrenia
   C. tumors and head trauma
   D. hypoglycemia and cerebrovascular disease
   E. drug and alcohol withdrawal

3. Sudden, excessive neuronal firing associated with

   seizures is inhibited by drugs that _____.
   A. inhibit dopamine synthesis and release
   B. delay the inflow of sodium ions and bind to T-type calcium channels
   C. inhibit serotonin reuptake
   D. inhibit acetylcholine

4. Which symptom is *not* associated with grand mal

   seizures? _____
   A. Convulsions
   B. Brief vacant stare
   C. Jerking movements
   D. Difficulty breathing

5. A grand mal seizure is also known as

   _____.
   A. a petit mal seizure
   B. a tonic-clonic seizure
   C. status epilepticus
   D. a febrile seizure

6. Joe Sherman is taking Lamictal 25-mg tablets. Which of the following warnings should he be given?

   _____
   A. MAY CAUSE DROWSINESS OR DIZZINESS
   B. AVOID ALCOHOL
   C. AVOID SUNLIGHT
   D. TAKE ON AN EMPTY STOMACH
   E. A and B

7. Which drug can be prescribed for seizures and

   neuropathic pain? _____
   A. Dilantin
   B. Neurontin
   C. Depakote
   D. Zarontin

8. June Schultz is taking Depakote 250-mg delayed-release tablets. Which of the following warnings

   should she be given? _____
   A. MAY CAUSE DROWSINESS OR DIZZINESS
   B. TAKE WITH FOOD
   C. SWALLOW WHOLE; DO NOT CRUSH OR CHEW
   D. AVOID ALCOHOL
   E. All of the above

9. Pharmacy technicians should dispense the same

   manufacturer's formulation of _____
   each time a prescription is filled, if possible.
   A. lamotrigine
   B. topiramate
   C. phenytoin
   D. levetiracetam

1. What is the *generic name* for Dilantin? _____

2. What is the *generic name* for Depakote? _____

3. What is the *brand name* for fosphenytoin? _____

4. What is the *generic name* for Trileptal? _____

5. What is a *brand name* for carbamazepine? _____

6. What is a *brand name* for oxcarbazepine? _____

7. What is the *generic name* for Celontin? _____

8. What is the *brand name* for tiagabine? _____

9. What is the *generic name* for Lyrica (United States)? _____

10. What is the *generic name* for Sabril? _____

11. What is a *brand name* for ethosuximide? _____

12. What is the *brand name* for primidone? _____

13. What is the *generic name* for Valium? _____

14. What is the *brand name* for lacosamide? _____

15. What is a *brand name* for diazepam? _____

16. What is the *brand name* for levetiracetam? _____

17. What is the *generic name* for Topamax? _____

18. What is the *generic name* for Zonegran? _____

MATCHING

A. Characterized by brief periods of unconsciousness and vacant stares

B. Characterized by stiffened limbs, difficulty breathing, and jerking movements followed by disorientation and limpness

C. Medical emergency that results from repeated generalized seizures

D. Causes a person to experience unusual sensations or feelings

E. Characterized by jerking muscle movements and caused by contraction of major muscle groups

1. _____ Myoclonic seizure

2. _____ Status epilepticus

3. _____ Simple focal seizure

4. _____ Tonic-clonic seizure

5. _____ Absence seizure

MATCHING

Patient education is an essential component of therapeutics. Select the **best** warning label to apply to the prescription vial given to patients taking the drugs listed.

A. AVOID ANTACIDS
B. MAY BE HABIT FORMING
C. SHAKE WELL; DISCARD WITHIN 30 DAYS OF RECONSTITUTION
D. AVOID ALCOHOL

1. _____ Tegretol XR 200 mg

2. _____ Sabril 500-mg suspension

3. _____ phenytoin 50-mg chewable tablets

4. _____ Lyrica 300 mg

MATCHING

Match each drug to its mechanism of action.

A. Modulates ion channels
B. Blocks the reuptake of GABA
C. Increases inhibitory effects of GABA
D. Inhibits the enzyme that inactivates GABA
E. Inhibits the excitatory neurotransmitter glutamate

1. _____ Tegretol

2. _____ vigabatrin

3. _____ perampanel

4. _____ Depakote

5. _____ tiagabine

TRUE OR FALSE

1. _____ Status epilepticus must be treated with intravenous medications.

2. _____ Nearly 75% of all seizures have no known cause.

3. _____ The aim of pharmaceutical treatment of seizures is to suppress seizure activity.

4. _____ Carbamazepine should be protected from light and moisture.

5. _____ Flashing or strobe lights, such as those used in fire alarm systems, can trigger a seizure in susceptible individuals with epilepsy.

6. _____ Depakote sprinkles must be swallowed whole.

7. _____ Most children who have febrile seizures will develop epilepsy.

8. _____ Gabapentin produces its effects by binding to $GABA_A$ receptors.

9. _____ There are only a few medications indicated to treat absence seizures.

10. _____ One serious side effect of phenobarbital is respiratory depression.

11. _____ Rectal diazepam may be used daily if needed.

12. _____ People with epilepsy have abnormally high levels of excitatory neurotransmitters and low levels of inhibitory neurotransmitters.

53

The following hard copies are brought to your pharmacy for filling. Identify the prescription error(s). (You already have the patient's full address on file.) There may be one error, more than one error, or no errors at all.

Micheal Vessalago, MD Date _____
1221 Madison #310
Anytown, USA

Pt. Name _____ Mary Smith _____
Address _____

℞ Topamax 200mg
    1 BID

Refills __11__

_____Vessalago_____
Substitution permitted   Dispense as written

---

1. Spot the error in the following prescription:

_____

A. Quantity missing
B. Strength missing
C. Strength incorrect
D. Directions missing
E. Dosage form incorrect

Anh Dang Tu, MD Date _____
1145 Broadway
Anytown, USA

Pt. Name _____ Lili Ng _____
Address _____

℞ phenytoin 10.0mg cap   #90
    1 cap TID for epilepsy

Refills _____

_____Tu_____
Substitution permitted   Dispense as written

---

2. Spot the error in the following prescription:

_____

A. Quantity missing
B. Directions incomplete
C. Strength missing
D. Strength incorrect
E. Dosage form incorrect

Marc Cordova, MD Date _____
1145 Broadway
Anytown, USA

Pt. Name _____ Sheila Wellcome _____
Address _____

℞ Neurontin 600mg cap   #90
    1 cap TID

Refills _____

_____Cordova_____
Substitution permitted   Dispense as written

---

3. Spot the error in the following prescription:

_____

A. Quantity missing
B. Directions incomplete
C. Strength missing
D. Strength incorrect
E. Dosage form incorrect

4. List two pairs of drug names that have look-alike or sound-alike issues with drugs used to treat seizure disorders.

DRUG NAME	LOOK-ALIKE OR SOUND-ALIKE DRUG

5. Susan Heller has been diagnosed with epilepsy and prescribed Keppra, 500 mg 1 BID, increased by 500 mg per dose every 2 weeks, until she is taking 3 g daily. For approximately how many days will 200 tablets last? Please show your calculations.

_____

_____

_____

_____

6. You receive a prescription from Sheila Harper for Trileptal to treat epilepsy. Sheila weighs 60 pounds. If Sheila should receive 9 mg/kg/day, approximately how many milligrams of Trileptal should she take every day? Please show your calculations.

_____

_____

_____

_____

_____

7. Adolescents treated for status epilepticus with lorazepam should receive 0.07 mg/kg/dose over 2 to 5 minutes (not more than 4 mg in a single dose); the dose may be repeated in 10 to 15 minutes. If Billy weighs 117 pounds, what dose should he be administered? Is this dose within the normal range? Please show your calculations.

_____

_____

_____

_____

_____

1. Concussions and other traumatic brain injuries have been a growing concern lately, especially in children. Research the association between concussion, traumatic brain injury, and seizures at https://mnepilepsy.org/news/concussion-traumatic-brain-injury-and-seizures/. Should patients with a traumatic brain injury be put on anti-seizure medications as prophylaxis? Why or why not?

_____

_____

_____

_____

CASE STUDY

Tyler is an adolescent male admitted to your hospital for seizures. His seizures are not characterized by convulsions or twitching, but instead he has been having episodes where he is unresponsive and staring off into space.

1. What type of seizures has Tyler been experiencing?

_____

2. Describe the role that neurotransmitters, specifically GABA and glutamate, have in epilepsy.

_____

_____

_____

_____

_____

Tyler has had numerous generalized seizures over a short time period, and his doctors have determined he has progressed into status epilepticus. He has already been given IV diazepam, and now his doctor has ordered fosphenytoin.

3. Describe how fosphenytoin will be administered.

_____

_____

_____

_____

At discharge, Tyler's doctor would like to start him on a new medication to treat and prevent his seizures.

4. List three medications that are indicated for the type of seizure Tyler has been experiencing.

_____

_____

_____

5. Tyler's doctor wrote a prescription for Depakote. Tyler expresses that he does not like swallowing large pills. What is a dosage form you could choose to dispense, and how would Tyler be instructed to use it?

_____

_____

_____

_____

_____

10 Treatment of Pain and Migraine Headache

TERMS AND DEFINITIONS

Match each term with the correct definition below.

A. Acute pain
B. Acupuncture
C. Analgesic
D. Arthritis
E. Biofeedback
F. Breakthrough pain
G. Cephalgia
H. Chronic pain
I. Cluster headache
J. Diabetic neuropathy
K. Dysphoria
L. Endorphins
M. Euphoria
N. Hyperalgesia
O. Inflammation
P. Migraine
Q. Neuropathic pain
R. Nociceptors
S. NSAID
T. Opiate naïve
U. Opioid
V. PCA
W. Plasticity
X. Shingles
Y. Substance P
Z. Trigeminal neuralgia

1. _____ are thin nerve fibers in skin, muscle, and other body tissues that carry pain signals.

2. _____ is a disorder that occurs in people with diabetes and causes numbness, pain, or tingling in the feet or legs.

3. A drug that reduces pain is called a(n) _____.

4. Naturally occurring or synthetically derived _____ analgesics have properties similar to those of morphine.

5. Sudden pain or _____ that results from injury or inflammation is usually self-limiting.

6. _____ is a response to tissue irritation or injury that is marked by signs of redness, swelling, heat, and pain.

7. _____ is a procedure that involves the application of needles to precise points on the body.

8. Pain that persists for a long period of time that is worsened by psychological factors and is resistant to many medical treatments is classified as _____.

9. _____ is a condition that is associated with joint pain.

10. Painful skin rash associated with _____ is caused by the reactivation of the herpes zoster virus.

11. The peptide that is involved in the production of pain sensations and that controls pain perception is called _____.

12. _____, enkephalins and dynorphins are natural painkillers.

13. _____ is a painful condition that produces intense, stabbing pain in areas of the face innervated by branches of the trigeminal nerve.

14. _____ is a feeling of emotional and/or mental discomfort, restlessness, and depression and is the opposite of _____.

15. _____ involves relaxation techniques and the gaining of self-control over muscle tension, heart rate, and skin temperature.

16. The ability of the brain to restructure itself and adapt to injury is called _____.

17. A type of pain that is associated with nerve injury, called _____, may be caused by trauma, infection, or chronic diseases such as diabetes.

18. _____ is pain that occurs between scheduled doses of analgesics.

19. _____ is head pain.

20. _____ is intensely painful vascular headache that occurs in groups and produces pain on one side of the head.

21. _____ is heightened sensitivity to pain that can result from treatment of chronic pain with high-dose opioids.

22. A _____ is a vascular headache that is often accompanied by nausea and visual disturbances.

23. _____ is the acronym for nonsteroidal anti-inflammatory drug.

24. Buprenorphine will have an agonist effect in patients who are _____.

25. Using a device connected to a patient's IV line, the patient can push a button to deliver a dose of pain medication using _____.

MULTIPLE CHOICE

1. Duragesic patches should be replaced every _____ hours.
   A. 12
   B. 24
   C. 36
   D. 72

2. Buprenorphine tablets _____.
   A. may be prescribed by any licensed prescriber
   B. may be prescribed for the treatment of opioid dependence only by specially licensed and authorized prescribers
   C. are available in combination with naltrexone by the trade name Suboxone (United States)
   D. may cause excitation

3. If a patient has received too much Sublimaze in the operating room, which narcotic antagonist should be available to reverse respiratory depression? _____
   A. diphenoxylate atropine
   B. naltrexone
   C. acetaminophen with codeine no. 4
   D. naloxone

4. The mu opioid receptor is known to cause which effects when activated? _____
   A. Decreased GI motility
   B. Respiratory depression
   C. Physical dependence
   D. Analgesia
   E. All of the above

Chapter **10 Treatment of Pain and Migraine Headache**

5. Which of the following two agents might be used to treat opioid-dependent patients? _____
   A. fentanyl and naltrexone
   B. methadone and hydrocodone
   C. Stadol and oxycodone
   D. Suboxone and naltrexone

6. Migraine prophylaxis can be initiated

   _____.
   A. When a patient must use sumatriptan more than three times per week
   B. Before trying acute agents such as Tylenol No. 3
   C. When a patient has six or more migraines per month
   D. In very few cases, as no drug has been shown to help

7. Select the statement that is true:
   A. Mixed opioids act like an agonist in patients who are currently taking meperidine.
   B. Naltrexone usually won't precipitate withdrawal symptoms when given to a patient who is dependent on opioids.
   C. Short-acting opioids are used for breakthrough pain.
   D. The use of fentanyl and hydrocodone is reserved for the management of drug dependence.

8. Which of these drugs is an opioid antagonist?

   _____
   A. oxycodone
   B. Vicodin
   C. ReVia
   D. Dolophine

9. NSAIDs can cause all of the following side effects

   except _____.
   A. Decreased blood pressure
   B. GI ulcers
   C. Fluid retention
   D. Agranulocytosis

FILL IN THE BLANK: DRUG NAMES

1. What is the *brand name* for hydrocodone and ibuprofen? _____

2. What is the *generic name* for Tylenol with Codeine No. 4? _____

3. What is the *generic name* for Dilaudid? _____

4. What is the *generic name* for Suboxone? _____

5. What is the *brand name* for naproxen? _____

6. What is the *generic name* for Anexsia (United States)? _____

7. What is the *brand name* for indomethacin? _____

8. What are *brand name*s for sustained-release morphine? _____and

   _____

9. What is a *brand name* for meperidine? _____

10. What is the *generic name* for Toradol? _____

11. What is the *generic name* for Imitrex? _____

12. What is a *brand name* for buprenorphine? _____

13. What is the *brand name* for buprenorphine plus naloxone? _____

14. What is the *generic name* for Stadol? _____

15. What is the *brand name* for eletriptan? _____

MATCHING

Patient education is an essential component of therapeutics. Select the **best** warning label to apply to the prescription vial given to patients taking the drugs listed.

A. DO NOT EXCEED
   RECOMMENDED DOSAGE
B. DO NOT INJECT MORE THAN
   2 DOSES IN 24 HOURS
C. AVOID ASPIRIN AND
   RELATED DRUGS

1. _____ Clinoril

2. _____ Maxalt

3. _____ Imitrex subcut

MATCHING

Match each drug to its pharmacological classification.

A. Opioid agonist
B. *Ergot alkaloids*
C. Triptan
D. Beta blocker

1. _____ Duragesic

2. _____ DHE

3. _____ Frova

4. _____ Inderal

TRUE OR FALSE

1. _____ Opiate naïve means without knowledge or understanding of the use of painkillers.

2. _____ Duragesic patches should be dispensed with instructions on proper storage and disposal to prevent accidental poisoning.

3. _____ Patient-controlled analgesia increases the patient's anxiety associated with pain.

4. _____ Patient-controlled analgesia permits patients to control the frequency of administration of their dose of pain medications.

5. _____ Endorphins, enkephalins, and dynorphin are substances that are released by the body in response to painful stimuli and that act as natural painkillers.

6. _____ Biofeedback and acupuncture are nonpharmacological treatments for pain.

7. _____ The peptide that is involved in the production of pain sensations and that controls pain perception is called substance X.

8. _____ Celebrex is the only remaining COX-2 inhibitor marketed in the United States and Canada.

The following hard copies are brought to your pharmacy for filling. Identify the prescription error(s). (You already have the patient's full address on file.) There may be one error, more than one error, or no errors at all.

Kathy Principi, MD   Date _____
1145 Broadway
Anytown, USA

Pt. Name _____ Sheila Wilcox _____
Address _____

℞ Duragesic 25mcg   #5
     1 patch daily

Refills _____
_____ Principi _____   _____
Substitution permitted   Dispense as written

---

1. Spot the error in the following prescription:

   _____

   A. Quantity missing
   B. Strength missing
   C. Strength incorrect
   D. Directions incorrect
   E. Dosage form incorrect

Kathy Principi, MD   Date _____
1145 Broadway
Anytown, USA

Pt. Name _____ Ellen Wilber _____
Address _____

℞ Stadol 10mg/ml   1 bottle
     1 spray in each nostril repeat when needed

Refills _____
_____ Principi _____   _____
Substitution permitted   Dispense as written

---

2. Spot the error in the following prescription:

   _____

   A. Quantity missing
   B. Directions incorrect
   C. Strength missing
   D. Strength incorrect
   E. Dosage form incorrect

Marc Cordova, MD   Date _____
1145 Broadway
Anytown, USA

Pt. Name _____ Alvin Sorrento _____
Address _____

℞ hydrocodone 5mg/acetaminophen 500mg tab
     i tab q 4-6h

Refills _____
_____ Cordova _____   _____
Substitution permitted   Dispense as written

---

3. Spot the error in the following prescription:

   _____

   A. Quantity missing
   B. Strength missing
   C. Strength incorrect
   D. Directions incorrect
   E. Dosage form incorrect

4. List four pairs of drug names that have look-alike or sound-alike issues with drugs used to treat pain.

DRUG NAME	LOOK-ALIKE OR SOUND-ALIKE DRUG

5. Nick Harper has been prescribed a pain "cocktail" containing Dolophine, 10 mg/5 mL, and hydroxyzine HCl, 50 mg/5 mL, in cherry syrup. He is instructed to take 1 teaspoonful every 6 hours. How many Dolophine tablets must you use to prepare 150 mL of the pain cocktail? (You will be using Dolophine 5-mg tablets.) Please show your calculations.

_____

_____

_____

_____

_____

6. If Mr. Strong is admitted to the hospital and administered Buprenex, how much will you draw up in the syringe for a 0.6-mg dose? How many milliliters (mL) will be needed per day if the dosage range is 0.3 to 0.6 mg every 6 hours? (Buprenex 0.3 mg/mL.) Please show your calculations.

_____

_____

_____

_____

_____

RESEARCH ACTIVITY

1. The fear of prescribing, dispensing, or taking opioid pain medications is called *opiophobia*. Use the Internet to research controlled substances. Locate treatment guidelines for terminal illness. When are concerns warranted? When are concerns not warranted?

_____

_____

_____

_____

_____

CASE STUDY

Dan is a 45-year-old male who fell from an 8-foot ladder while cleaning his gutters. He injured his back as a result of his fall. His doctor has prescribed meloxicam and hydrocodone/acetaminophen for his pain.

1. Explain why the doctor would choose meloxicam to treat Dan's pain. (Hint: What is the pharmacologic class of meloxicam?)

   _____

   _____

   _____

   _____

2. Describe the role of cytokines, prostaglandins, and other mediators of pain in inflammation.

   _____

   _____

   _____

   _____

One year later, you notice that Dan has been filling his hydrocodone/acetaminophen prescription more frequently than before. He explains to you that his low back pain has spread to pain in his legs and that he has needed to use more of his medication to control his pain.

3. Hydrocodone/acetaminophen is an opioid agonist. Describe the effects produced by mu receptor activation by opioid agonists.

   _____

   _____

   _____

   _____

4. Compare and contrast tolerance and dependence.

   _____

   _____

   _____

   _____

5. Treating chronic pain requires a multimodal approach. Explain what this means, and list some nondrug therapies you could suggest to Dan to help manage his pain.

_____

_____

_____

_____

_____

11 Treatment of Sleep Disorders and Attention-Deficit Hyperactivity Disorder

TERMS AND DEFINITIONS

Match each term with the correct definition below.

A. Hypnotic
B. Insomnia
C. Melatonin
D. Non–REM sleep
E. Rapid eye movement sleep
F. Rebound hypersomnia
G. Sedative
H. Stimulant

1. _____ is a hormone released by the pineal gland that regulates body temperature, helps regulate our circadian rhythm, and makes us feel drowsy.

2. _____, or excessive sleep, is an adverse effect associated with long-term use of drugs that depress rapid eye movement (REM) and non–REM sleep.

3. A drug that increases activity in the brain is called a(n)

   _____ and can be used to treat attention-deficit/hyperactivity disorder (ADHD) and narcolepsy.

4. A _____ is a drug that is used to treat _____, a condition characterized by difficulty in falling asleep and/or staying asleep.

5. A _____ is a medication that causes relaxation and promotes drowsiness.

6. The stages of sleep are categorized as _____ and

   _____.

MULTIPLE CHOICE

1. Sleep deprivation is linked to all of the following

   except _____.
   A. increased illness
   B. motor vehicle accidents
   C. increased mental agility
   D. lack of productivity

2. Patient GL has been diagnosed with narcolepsy and has been prescribed Provigil. GL is also taking Tylenol for headaches, Imitrex for migraines, Neurontin for nerve pain, and Sprintec for birth control. Of these four medications, which one has the most pressing interaction with Provigil?
   A. Tylenol
   B. Imitrex
   C. Neurontin
   D. Sprintec

3. Which of the following is *not* linked to insomnia?

_____
A. Sleep apnea
B. Use of depressant drugs
C. Consumption of caffeinated beverages and foods
D. Use of stimulant drugs
E. Chronic pain and illness

4. Select the advice that would *not* be a tip to prevent

insomnia. _____.
A. Avoid stimulants close to bedtime.
B. Adopt a regular sleeping schedule.
C. Take daytime naps.
D. Exercise.
E. Do not lie in bed awake.

5. Prescription drugs used to treat insomnia are

_____.
A. benzodiazepine receptor agonists and benzodiazepines
B. decongestants and analgesics
C. NSAIDs and antibiotics
D. barbiturates and decongestants

6. Homer Street calls the pharmacy to renew his "sleeping pill." His profile shows he has recently taken the drugs listed below. Which drug is the

"sleeping pill"? _____
A. Buspirone
B. Alprazolam
C. Triazolam
D. Fluoxetine

7. The pharmacist reminds Mr. Street to avoid

concurrent use of _____ when he takes his "sleeping pill."
A. ASA
B. antacids
C. APAP
D. alcohol

8. Pharmaceutical treatment of ADHD is achieved with the administration of all of the following *except*

_____.
A. temazepam
B. methylphenidate
C. Adderall
D. Concerta

9. A patient comes into the pharmacy complaining of recent insomnia. What is something he can try before beginning pharmacological treatment?
A. Have a small snack before bed to avoid going to bed hungry.
B. If he can't fall asleep quickly, he should simply lie in bed until he can.
C. Exercise 1 to 2 hours before bedtime.
D. Drink a cup of coffee with dinner.

10. Which warning label should *not* be affixed to prescription vials for Adderall XR?

_____
A. TAKE WITH FOOD
B. MAY BE HABIT FORMING
C. SWALLOW WHOLE; DO NOT CRUSH OR CHEW
D. MAY CAUSE DROWSINESS

FILL IN THE BLANK: DRUG NAMES

1. What is the **brand name** for doxepin? _____

2. What is the **generic name** for Unisom? _____

3. What is a **brand name** for armodafinil? _____

4. What is the **generic name** for Dalmane? _____

5. What is the **generic name** for Restoril? _____

6. What is the **generic name** for Halcion? _____

7. What is the **generic name** for Lunesta (United States)? _____

8. What is the **generic name** for Sonata (United States) and Starnoc (Canada)? _____

9. What is the **generic name** for Ambien (United States)? _____

10. What is the **generic name** for Imovane (Canada)? _____

Chapter **11** **Treatment of Sleep Disorders and Attention-Deficit Hyperactivity Disorder**

11. What is the **brand name** for amphetamine plus dextroamphetamine? _____

12. What is the **generic name** for Provigil (United States)? _____

13. What is the **brand name** for dextroamphetamine? _____

14. What are **brand names** for methylphenidate? _____

15. What is the **brand name** for atomoxetine? _____

MATCHING

Match each drug to its pharmacological classification.

A. melatonin agonist
B. benzodiazepine
C. amphetamine
D. nonamphetamine stimulant

1. _____ Strattera

2. _____ Vyvanse

3. _____ Halcion

4. _____ Ramelteon

TRUE OR FALSE

1. _____ Rapid eye movement sleep is the stage of sleep where dreaming occurs.

2. _____ Pharmacological treatment for insomnia is recommended for long-term therapy.

3. _____ Our normal sleep-wake cycle is linked to changes in sunlight.

4. _____ Melatonin and valerian root are natural remedies that have proven effectiveness for promoting sleep.

5. _____ Benzodiazepines provide an effective treatment option for patients with narcolepsy.

CRITICAL THINKING

The following hard copies are brought to your pharmacy for filling. Identify the prescription error(s). (You already have the patient's full address on file.) There may be one error, more than one error, or no errors at all.

Micheal Vessalago, MD   Date _____
1221 Madison #310
Anytown, USA

Pt. Name _____ Bart Klitgaard _____

Address _____

℞ secobarbital 100mg caps   #10
      iHS

Refills   2

Vessalago   AV1111119   _____

Substitution permitted   Dispense as written

1. Spot the error in the following prescription:

   _____

   A. Quantity missing

   B. RF limit exceeded

   C. Strength missing

   D. Strength incorrect

   E. Dosage form incorrect

```
┌─────────────────────────────────────────┐
│         Marc Cordova, MD      Date _____ │
│           1145 Broadway                   │
│           Anytown, USA                    │
│  Pt. Name _____ Crystal Boelle _____  │
│  Address _____  │
│  ℞  triazolam 0.25mg                      │
│       i tab at bedtime                    │
│                                           │
│                                           │
│  Refills _____                           │
│                            Cordova        │
│  _____    _____  │
│  Substitution permitted  Dispense as written │
└─────────────────────────────────────────┘
```

2. Spot the error in the following prescription:
   _____

   A. Quantity missing
   B. RF limit exceeded
   C. Strength missing
   D. Strength incorrect
   E. Dosage form incorrect

3. List two pairs of drug names that have look-alike or sound-alike issues with drugs used to treat sleep disorders and those used to treat ADHD.

DRUG NAME	LOOK-ALIKE OR SOUND-ALIKE DRUG

RESEARCH ACTIVITY

1. Controversy exists with regard to the increasing numbers of diagnoses for ADHD and treatment for this disorder with stimulants. Do research on ADHD, and give reasons for and against treatment of it. Access the National Library of Medicine website (nlm.nih.gov/medlineplus/attentiondeficithyperactivitydisorder.html) or other websites to complete the research activity.

_____

_____

_____

_____

A patient comes into the pharmacy with a new prescription for zolpidem IR 10 mg. It's obvious that the patient is very drowsy and lethargic, and upon reviewing her chart, you notice that she's been taking this medication for 2 months with good adherence. When at the register, the patient says, "Maybe I shouldn't be taking this medication. I mean, it's clearly not working, I've only gotten four or five good nights of sleep since taking it! What other pills can I take to help me sleep?"

1. Before discussing other pharmacotherapy options, what are some questions you can ask this patient to assess her sleep hygiene? Write at least three questions.

_____

_____

_____

_____

2. The patient is worried about becoming dependent upon zolpidem. What are some medications for insomnia that are not controlled substances (in the United States?) What side effects might she experience with these medications?

_____

_____

_____

_____

A few months later, the patient comes back to the pharmacy to thank you for your advice regarding the treatment of insomnia. She is no longer taking zolpidem. She is pregnant and beginning to worry about her child getting ADHD.

3. What advice can you give this patient to reduce the risk of ADHD in her child?

_____

_____

_____

_____

_____

4. Would you tell her that following your advice listed above would eliminate any risk of her child getting ADHD? Why or why not?

_____

_____

_____

_____

_____

12 Neuromuscular Blockade and Muscle Spasms

TERMS AND DEFINITIONS

Match each term with the correct definition below.

A. Acetylcholinesterase
B. Amyotrophic lateral sclerosis
C. Anaphylactic shock
D. Botulinum toxin
E. Central-acting muscle relaxants
F. Cerebral palsy
G. Clonus
H. Depolarizing neuromuscular blockers
I. Endotracheal intubation
J. End plate
K. Multiple sclerosis
L. Neuromuscular junction
M. Nondepolarizing competitive blockers
N. Peripheral-acting muscle relaxants
O. Sarcomere
P. Soleplate
Q. Spasticity
R. Tetanus

1. The space between the motor neuron end plate and the muscle soleplate that neurotransmitters must cross is called the _____.

2. _____ is the process of inserting a tube down into the trachea, or windpipe, to facilitate mechanical ventilation.

3. _____ is a condition that causes increased muscle tone and exaggerated motion.

4. Drugs that compete with acetylcholine for binding sites are called _____.

5. _____ is an autoimmune disorder characterized by the progressive destruction of the body's nerves.

6. A projection extending off the end of a motor neuron is called an _____ and is where the neurotransmitter acetylcholine is released.

7. _____ block nerve transmission between the motor end plate and skeletal muscle receptors.

8. The portion of the membrane of muscle cells that receives messages transmitted by motor neurons is called the _____.

9. The fatal condition _____ is characterized by continuous muscle spasm and is also known as "lockjaw."

10. Drugs that produce relaxation of muscles by central nervous system depression, blocking nerve transmission between the spinal cord and muscles, are called _____.

11. A poison produced by the bacterium *Clostridium botulinum*, _____, causes muscle paralysis.

12. An acute, life-threatening allergic reaction is also known as _____.

13. _____ produce sustained depolarization by causing acetylcholine receptor sites to convert to an inactive state.

14. An enzyme that degrades acetylcholine and reverses acetylcholine-induced depolarization is called _____.

15. _____ is more commonly known as Lou Gehrig's disease.

16. _____ is a neurological disorder that affects muscle movement and coordination.

17. The _____ is the contracting unit of muscle fibers.

18. Involuntary rhythmic muscle contraction, called _____ , causes the feet and wrists to involuntarily flex and relax.

MULTIPLE CHOICE

1. Depolarizing neuromuscular blockers produce sustained depolarization by causing

   _____ receptor sites to convert to an inactive state.
   A. norepinephrine
   B. dopamine
   C. GABA
   D. acetylcholine

2. Which symptom is *not* associated with anaphylactic

   shock? _____
   A. Peripheral vasodilation
   B. Bradycardia
   C. Bronchospasm
   D. Laryngeal edema
   E. Airway obstruction

3. Neuromuscular blocking drugs are classified as

   "_____" by the Interdisciplinary Safe Medication Use Expert Committee of the United States Pharmacopoeia.
   A. dangerous
   B. high alert
   C. low alert
   D. use with caution

4. Select the drug that reverses the effects of

   neuromuscular blocking agents. _____
   A. vecuronium
   B. rocuronium
   C. neostigmine
   D. mivacurium
   E. pancuronium

5. According to the Interdisciplinary Safe Medication Use Expert Committee of the United States

   Pharmacopoeia, the warning label _____ should always be placed on dispensed neuromuscular blocking drugs.
   A. KEEP IN REFRIGERATOR
   B. WARNING: PARALYZING AGENT
   C. WARNING: ALLERGIC REACTIONS POSSIBLE
   D. FOR ONETIME USE ONLY

6. Which of the following is true about the use of neuromuscular blocking agents?
   A. Neuromuscular blocking drugs are delivered parenterally due to poor absorption when taken orally.
   B. Neuromuscular blockers are generally safe and do not require any extra precautions for safety.
   C. They are commonly used when patients have an acute anxiety attack.
   D. None of the above are true.

7. Botox injections can cause all of the following

   adverse reactions *except* _____.
   A. droopy eyelid muscles
   B. headache
   C. muscle weakness
   D. drowsiness
   E. flulike syndrome

Chapter **12 Neuromuscular Blockade and Muscle Spasms**

8. Which drug is used for the treatment of muscle strain? _____
   A. carisoprodol
   B. diazepam
   C. dantrolene
   D. baclofen

9. Which of the muscle relaxants listed can discolor urine? _____
   A. diazepam
   B. chlorzoxazone
   C. methocarbamol
   D. B and C

FILL IN THE BLANK: DRUG NAMES

1. What is the **brand name** for succinylcholine? _____

2. What is the **generic name** for Botox? _____

3. What is the **generic name** for Nimbex? _____

4. What is the **generic name** for Dantrium? _____

5. What is the **brand name** for rocuronium? _____

6. What is the **generic name** for Zanaflex? _____

7. What is the **brand name** for pyridostigmine? _____

MATCHING

A. Depolarizing neuromuscular blockers

B. Nondepolarizing neuromuscular blockers

C. Neuromuscular blockade reversal agent

1. succinylcholine _____

2. onabotulinumtoxin A _____

3. pyridostigmine _____

TRUE OR FALSE

1. _____ Acetylcholinesterase is an enzyme that reverses acetylcholine-induced depolarization by degrading acetylcholine.

2. _____ Botox is known to cause side effects such as droopy eyelids, headache, nausea, and muscle weakness

3. _____ The onset of action of neuromuscular blocking drugs is slow (1–2 hours) and the duration of action is long (12–24 hours)

4. _____ The endings -*curonium* and -*curium* are commonly used for nondepolarizing neuromuscular blockers.

5. _____ Look-alike packaging is a problem that can be attributed to drug manufacturers as well as to pharmacies dispensing drugs.

6. _____ Skeletal muscle relaxants should be used along with nonpharmaceutical therapies such as rest, exercise, cryotherapy, and physical therapy.

7. _____ There are five phases in the development of spasticity.

1. List two pairs of drug names that have look-alike or sound-alike issues with drugs used for neuromuscular blockade.

DRUG NAME	LOOK-ALIKE OR SOUND-ALIKE DRUG

RESEARCH ACTIVITY

1. What causes tetanus, and how is the disorder managed? Check the *Merck Manual* website (http://www.merckmanuals.com/professional) and other websites to complete the research activity.

_____

_____

_____

_____

CASE STUDY

You are working in a small hospital as a pharmacy technician. The number of surgeries and intubations at the hospital is increasing, so the pharmacy manager decides to start carrying more neuromuscular blockers in the pharmacy. To keep things organized, the manager wants to store all of the neuromuscular blockers on a single shelf.

1. What advice can you offer the pharmacy manager about the proper storage of neuromuscular blocking agents? Provide at least three examples.

_____

_____

_____

_____

2. As a pharmacy technician, what are some key administration pieces of information to remember when you are dispensing a neuromuscular blocking agent?

_____

_____

_____

_____

13 Treatment of Gout, Osteoarthritis, and Rheumatoid Arthritis

TERMS AND DEFINITIONS

Match each term with the correct definition below.

A. Arthritis
B. Autoimmune disease
C. Autoantibody
D. Gout
E. Hyperuricemia
F. Rheumatoid arthritis
G. Rheumatoid factor
H. Synovium
I. Tumor necrosis factor
J. Urates
K. Uricosuric

1. The immunoglobulin (antibody) _____ is present in many people who have _____, a chronic disease characterized by inflammation of the joints.

2. _____ is a condition characterized by increased levels of urates in the blood.

3. A disease that occurs when the immune system turns against the parts of the body it is designed to protect is called an _____.

4. _____ is an inflammatory condition that produces joint pain.

5. The _____ is a thin layer of tissue that lines the joint space.

6. The term used to describe an abnormal antibody that attacks healthy cells and tissues is _____.

7. _____ is a disease characterized by joint deposits of urate crystals.

8. The inflammatory cytokine found in the synovial fluid of rheumatoid arthritis patients is called _____.

9. A drug that increases the body's clearance of urates is referred to as _____.

10. _____ is/are the product of purine metabolism.

1. Hyperuricemia is associated with all of the

   following conditions *except* _____.
   A. Coronary heart disease and stroke
   B. Diabetes and insulin resistance
   C. Rheumatoid arthritis
   D. Kidney disease
   E. Hypertension

2. Which of the following is a joint commonly affected

   by gout? _____
   A. Big toe
   B. Ankle
   C. Knee
   D. Wrist
   E. All of the above

3. Which drug blocks the final enzymatic step in the

   production of uric acid? _____
   A. colchicine
   B. probenecid
   C. allopurinol
   D. hydrochlorothiazide
   E. celecoxib

4. Which foods and beverages are most likely to
   increase the risk of a gout attack?

   _____
   A. Seafood such as anchovies, herring, mussels, or
      trout
   B. Seafood such as crab, lobster, oysters, or shrimp
   C. Meats such as beef, duck, chicken, or pork
   D. Dairy such as skim milk and cheese

5. Select the warning label that should *not* be applied
   to prescriptions for cyclosporine oral solution.

   _____
   A. DO NOT REFRIGERATE
   B. PROTECT FROM LIGHT
   C. DILUTE SOLUTION AND USE
      IMMEDIATELY
   D. REFRIGERATE; DO NOT FREEZE

6. Cyclosporine parenteral solution is stable for

   _____ hours in normal saline glass
   bottles.
   A. 6
   B. 9
   C. 12
   D. 24

7. Which of the following statements regarding the
   progression of rheumatoid arthritis is false?

   _____
   A. Swelling, pain, and stiffness begin in phase 1,
      when the synovium becomes inflamed.
   B. In phase 2, rapid cell death causes the synovium
      to become thinner.
   C. Pain and disability increase in phase 3 as
      enzymes digest bone and cartilage.
   D. RA can cause other symptoms such as fatigue,
      weakness, muscle pain, decreased appetite, and
      depression.

8. Which of the following is **not** an adverse effect of

   glucocorticoids? _____
   A. hypoglycemia
   B. insomnia
   C. weight gain
   D. euphoria

9. Select the **true** statement. _____
   A. Biological response modifiers stimulate the
      release of cells that mobilize to fight what the
      body believes is a harmful invasion.
   B. Biological response modifiers interfere with the
      activity of cytokines, leukocytes, B cells, and T
      cells.
   C. Selective COX-2 inhibitors decrease the risk for
      cardiovascular toxicity and gastrointestinal
      ulceration.
   D. Tumor necrosis factor-alpha inhibitors are
      produced by the body and block the
      inflammatory process.

10. Gold compounds are used in the treatment of

    _____.
    A. rheumatoid arthritis
    B. multiple sclerosis
    C. myositis
    D. systemic lupus erythematosus

11. Which drug is *not* used for the treatment of
    rheumatoid arthritis?
    A. Remicade
    B. gold salts
    C. leflunomide
    D. dantrolene
    E. penicillamine

FILL IN THE BLANK: DRUG NAMES

1. What is the *brand name* for colchicine? _____

2. What is the *generic name* for Krystexxa? _____

3. What is the *brand name* for febuxostat? _____

4. What is a *brand name* for prednisolone? _____

5. What is the *generic name* for Cortef? _____

6. What is a *brand name* for celecoxib? _____

7. What is the *generic name* for Medrol? _____

8. What is the *brand name* for hydroxychloroquine? _____

9. What is the *generic name* for Imuran? _____

10. What is a *brand name* for etanercept? _____

11. What is the *generic name* for Sandimmune and Neoral? _____

12. What is a *brand name* for adalimumab? _____

13. What is the *brand name* for infliximab? _____

14. What is the *brand name* for anakinra? _____

15. What is the *brand name* for leflunomide? _____

16. What is a *brand name* for auranofin? _____

17. What is the *generic name* for Cuprimine and Depen? _____

MATCHING

Patient education is an essential component of therapeutics. Select the **best** warning label to apply to the prescription vial given to patients taking the drugs listed.

A. TAKE ON AN EMPTY STOMACH

B. AVOID GRAPEFRUIT JUICE

C. AVOID ASPIRIN

D. AVOID PROLONGED EXPOSURE TO SUNLIGHT

E. MAY CAUSE DIZZINESS OR DROWSINESS

1. _____ cyclosporine oral solution

2. _____ allopurinol

3. _____ probenecid

4. _____ hydroxychloroquine

5. _____ penicillamine

TRUE OR FALSE

1. _____ Probenecid and allopurinol should be taken on an empty stomach.

2. _____ Colchicine is a uricosuric.

3. _____ Osteoarthritis is the most common of all arthritic conditions.

4. _____ The presence of rheumatoid factor in a patient is a definitive sign that the patient has rheumatoid arthritis.

5. _____ The reconstituted solution of azathioprine must be shaken vigorously.

6. _____ The pharmacy should try to dispense the same manufacturer's product of cyclosporine each time the prescription is refilled.

7. _____ Rheumatoid arthritis is far more common in men than in women.

8. _____ Celecoxib is the only selective COX-2 inhibitor still available for use in the United States and Canada.

CRITICAL THINKING

The following hard copies are brought to your pharmacy for filling. Identify the prescription error(s). (You already have the patient's full address on file.) There may be one error, more than one error, or no errors at all.

Kathy Principi, MD   Date _____
1145 Broadway
Anytown, USA
Pt. Name _____ Barry Wilcox _____
Address _____
Rx Celebrex 200mg tablets   #30
i tab daily
Refills _____
_____ Principi _____
Substitution permitted   Dispense as written

1. Spot the error in the following prescription:

   _____

   A. Quantity missing

   B. Strength missing

   C. Strength incorrect

   D. Directions incorrect

   E. Dosage form incorrect

Kathy Principi, MD   Date _____
1145 Broadway
Anytown, USA
Pt. Name _____ Paulette Wilber _____
Address _____
Rx interferon β-1a   #4 prefilled syringes
inject 0.2ml SC every other day
Refills _____
_____ Principi _____
Substitution permitted   Dispense as written

2. Spot the error in the following prescription:

   _____

   A. Quantity missing

   B. Directions incorrect

   C. Strength missing

   D. Strength incorrect

   E. Dosage form incorrect

Chapter **13** **Treatment of Gout, Osteoarthritis, and Rheumatoid Arthritis**

3. List six pairs of drug names that have look-alike or sound-alike issues with drugs used to treat muscle spasms.

DRUG NAME	LOOK-ALIKE OR SOUND-ALIKE DRUG

RESEARCH ACTIVITY

1. Patients with gout will be advised to make lifestyle changes to reduce their risk for gout attacks. Check the National Library of Medicine website and other Internet sites to do research on gout and hyperuricemia (nlm.nih.gov/medlineplus/gout.html). Write a paragraph explaining what people with gout can do to stay healthy and avoid gout attacks.

_____

_____

_____

_____

2. Antibody testing provides an early screening test for some autoimmune diseases. Check the National Library of Medicine website (nlm.nih.gov/medlineplus/rheumatoidarthritis.html#cat1) and other Internet sites; then write a paragraph explaining the benefit of early diagnosis.

_____

_____

_____

_____

CASE STUDY

A familiar patient at the retail pharmacy where you work has been recently diagnosed with rheumatoid arthritis. She states that the doctor did not give her much information on her new disease; the doctor simply handed her a few new prescription pads and told her to schedule another appointment in 3 months. The patient is confused and asks for your help in her treatment for this disease.

1. In simple terms, describe the effects that rheumatoid arthritis has on the body. What is the difference between rheumatoid arthritis and arthritis?

   _____

   _____

   _____

   _____

2. The doctor gave the patient prescriptions for celecoxib, methotrexate, and Humira. How do each of these medications help in the treatment of RA? What is the onset of action for each of these three medications?

   _____

   _____

   _____

   _____

14 Treatment of Osteoporosis and Paget's Disease of the Bone

TERMS AND DEFINITIONS

Match each term with the correct definition below.

A. Bone mineral density
B. Bone resorption
C. Osteoblasts
D. Osteoclasts
E. Osteoporosis
F. Remodeling

1. _____ is a chronic, progressive disease of bone characterized by loss of bone density and increased risk for fractures.

2. The _____ test measures the degree of bone loss.

3. The term used to describe the process of continual turnover of bone is

   _____.

4. The process by which bone is broken down to mineral ions (calcium) is

   called _____.

5. _____ are cells responsible for bone formation, deposition, and mineralization of the collagen matrix of bone.

6. The cells responsible for bone resorption are called _____.

MULTIPLE CHOICE

1. The lifetime risk for fractures in women with

   osteoporosis is _____.
   A. 1 in 3
   B. 1 in 4
   C. 1 in 10
   D. 1 in 100

2. In a person with osteoporosis, a fragility fracture may

   occur when the person _____.
   A. falls
   B. coughs
   C. sneezes
   D. is in a car accident
   E. B and C

3. The percentage of total body calcium located in the

   skeleton is _____.
   A. 10%
   B. 50%
   C. 75%
   D. 99%
   E. 100%

4. Which hormone is *not* involved in the regulation of

   serum calcium levels? _____
   A. Parathyroid hormone
   B. Glucagon
   C. Calcitonin
   D. Vitamin D

5. _____ is a condition with the potential to cause secondary osteoporosis.
   A. Hypothyroidism
   B. Rheumatoid arthritis
   C. Inflammatory bowel disease
   D. All of the above

6. Which drug must be taken on an empty stomach at least 30 minutes before the first meal or beverage of the day? _____
   A. calcium
   B. Evista
   C. Fosamax
   D. Estrace

7. Patients taking Didronel and Actonel must sit upright or stand for at least _____ minutes after dosing to avoid possible esophageal ulceration.
   A. 30
   B. 60
   C. 90
   D. 120

8. What is the difference between calcium carbonate and calcium citrate supplements? _____
   A. Carbonate should be taken on an empty stomach, and citrate may be taken with or without food.
   B. Carbonate should be taken on a full stomach, and citrate may be taken with or without food.
   C. Carbonate provides the greatest amount of elemental calcium per tablet.
   D. B and C

9. The use of teriparatide, a genetically engineered form of human parathyroid hormone and the only drug currently available in this category, is limited because of risks for _____.
   A. fractures
   B. osteosarcoma
   C. pituitary tumors
   D. All of the above

FILL IN THE BLANK: DRUG NAMES

1. What is a **brand name** for pamidronate? _____

2. What is the **generic name** for Actonel? _____

3. What is a **brand name** for alendronate? _____

4. What is the **brand name** for etidronate? _____

5. What is the **generic name** for Zometa? _____

6. What is the **brand name** for raloxifene? _____

7. What is the **generic name** for Fosamax Plus D (United States)? _____

8. What is a **brand name(s)** for denosumab? _____

9. What is the **generic name** for Boniva? _____

10. What is the **generic name** for Climara? _____

11. What is the **brand name** for conjugated estrogens? _____

12. What is the **generic name** for Premphase and Prempro? _____

13. What is the **generic name** for Climara Pro? _____

14. What is the **generic name** for Ogen? _____

15. What is the **generic name** for Forteo (United States? _____

MATCHING

Patient education is an essential component of therapeutics. Select the **best** warning label to apply to the prescription vial given to patients taking the drugs listed.

A. ROTATE SITE OF APPLICATION
B. STORE IN MANUFACTURER'S SEALED FOIL POUCH
C. TAKE WITH FOOD
D. TAKE 30 MINUTES BEFORE THE FIRST MEAL OF THE DAY
E. TAKE WITH OR WITHOUT FOOD
F. TAKE 1 HOUR BEFORE THE FIRST MEAL OF THE DAY

1. _____ Actonel
2. _____ Climara
3. _____ Premarin
4. _____ CombiPatch
5. _____ Boniva
6. _____ Evista

MATCHING

Match each drug to its pharmacological classification.

A. monoclonal antibody
B. bisphosphonate
C. selective estrogen receptor modulator
D. estrogen replacement
E. anabolic agent

1. _____ Premarin
2. _____ Evista
3. _____ Forteo
4. _____ Fosamax
5. _____ Prolia

TRUE OR FALSE

1. _____ Denosumab binds to RANKL, resulting in an inhibition of osteoblast activation.

2. _____ Unlike Forteo, bisphosphonates cannot increase bone remodeling. They can only prevent further bone degradation.

3. _____ Some studies show that selective estrogen receptor modulators may increase the risk of esophageal cancer.

4. _____ If a patient is on levothyroxine, it's important to avoid calcium tablets within 30 minutes of taking the levothyroxine.

5. _____ Although Paget's disease of the bone and osteoporosis have different pathologies, they are treated similarly.

6. _____ Non–weight-bearing exercise such as swimming will help keep bones strong.

CRITICAL THINKING

The following hard copies are brought to your pharmacy for filling. Identify the prescription error(s). (You already have the patient's full address on file.) There may be one error, more than one error, or no errors at all.

```
Kathy Principi, MD        Date _____
1145 Broadway
Anytown, USA

Pt. Name _____ Belinda Wilcox _____
Address _____
Rx   Miacalcin nasal spray     1 bottle
     1 spray in each nostril daily



Refills _____
    Principi
_____        _____
Substitution permitted      Dispense as written
```

1. Spot the error in the following prescription:

   _____

   A. Quantity missing
   B. Strength missing
   C. Strength incorrect
   D. Directions incorrect
   E. Dosage form incorrect

```
Kathy Principi, MD        Date _____
1145 Broadway
Anytown, USA

Pt. Name _____ Paulette Wilber _____
Address _____
Rx   Fosamax 70mg once weekly




Refills _____
    Principi
_____        _____
Substitution permitted      Dispense as written
```

2. Spot the error in the following prescription:

   _____

   A. Quantity missing
   B. Directions incorrect
   C. Strength missing
   D. Strength incorrect
   E. Dosage form incorrect

3. List six pairs of drug names that have look-alike or sound-alike issues with drugs used to treat muscle spasms.

DRUG NAME	LOOK-ALIKE OR SOUND-ALIKE DRUG

RESEARCH ACTIVITY

1. Access the National Library of Medicine website (nlm.nih.gov/medlineplus/osteoporosis.html) and other Internet sites; then write a paragraph justifying the following recommendation: "It is best to lay the foundation for healthy dense bones early in life."

_____

_____

_____

_____

CASE STUDY

A 77-year-old female patient comes into the hospital with a broken wrist secondary to a fall. After a bone mineral density test, the doctor diagnoses the patient with osteoporosis. The pharmacist has assigned you to do a medication reconciliation on this patient.

1. Name at least five medications and five disease states that may be contributing to this patient's recently diagnosed condition.

_____

_____

_____

_____

2. Based on the patient's age, how much calcium does she need per day? What are three to five good sources of calcium that the patient may be able to add to her diet?

_____

_____

_____

_____

3. In your conversation with the patient, she tells you that she gets the majority of her exercise from swimming. Would you recommend any additional form of exercise for this patient? If so, what exercises would you recommend?

_____

_____

_____

_____

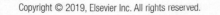
4. Research strategies to reduce falls in the patient's home using the following resource: https://www.ncoa.org/healthy-aging/falls-prevention/preventing-falls-tips-for-older-adults-and-caregivers/. Recommend three prevention steps she can take to prevent future falls.

_____

_____

_____

_____

Chapter **14** **Treatment of Osteoporosis and Paget's Disease of the Bone**

15 Treatment of Diseases of the Eye

TERMS AND DEFINITIONS

Match each term with the correct definition below.

A. Angle-closure glaucoma
B. Aqueous humor
C. Blepharitis
D. Conjunctivitis
E. Cytomegalovirus retinitis
F. Dry eye disease
G. Herpes simplex keratitis
H. Herpes zoster ophthalmicus
I. Intraocular pressure
J. Iritis
K. Keratitis
L. Open-angle glaucoma
M. Peripheral vision
N. Photopsia
O. Stye
P. Uveitis
Q. Vitreous floaters

1. _____ is a disorder characterized by elevated pressure in the eye; it can lead to permanent blindness.

2. Particles that float in the vitreous and appear as spots or spiders are referred to as _____.

3. _____ is a disease of the eye that results in the formation of scales on the eyelids and eyelashes.

4. _____ is a herpes virus infection of the eye characterized by excessive tearing, decreased vision, a gritty feeling in the eye, and pain when looking at bright light.

5. _____ is a condition associated with flashes of light.

6. The fluid that is made in the front part of the eye is called

_____.

7. Inflammation of the iris is referred to as _____.

8. _____ is sometimes called "side vision."

9. Blindness may occur as a result of _____, a painful herpes virus infection of the eye that causes a rash or sores around the eyes.

10. A _____ is a painful lump located on the eyelid margin caused by a self-limiting infection of the oil glands of the eyelid.

11. _____ is the pressure in the eye.

12. _____ is a condition that results from a lack of tears, whether due to lower production or faster evaporation.

13. _____ is characterized by a sudden increase in intraocular pressure caused by obstruction of the drainage portal between the cornea and the iris (angle).

14. _____, or more commonly known as pink eye, is a common ailment that produces itching and burning of the eye.

15. _____ is an opportunistic infection of the eye that occurs in patients who have HIV/AIDS or who take immunosuppressive drugs.

16. A severe infection of the cornea that may be caused by bacteria or fungi is called _____.

17. _____ is a serious eye condition that produces inflammation of the uvea and can cause scarring of the eye and blindness if untreated.

MULTIPLE CHOICE

1. _____ is usually the first area of vision to be lost with glaucoma.
   A. Peripheral vision
   B. Near vision
   C. Far vision
   D. Central vision

2. Carbonic anhydrase inhibitors may cause allergic reactions in people who have allergies to _____ anti-infective agents.
   A. penicillin
   B. tetracycline
   C. sulfonamide
   D. macrolide

3. Adverse effects of alpha agonists include _____.
   A. Dry eyes
   B. Decreased night vision
   C. Blurred vision
   D. All of the above

4. The mechanism of action for drugs used in the treatment of glaucoma is _____.
   A. to increase the formation of aqueous humor
   B. to decrease the formation of aqueous humor
   C. to promote the drainage of aqueous humor
   D. to decrease the drainage of aqueous humor
   E. B and C

5. All of the following drug classifications decrease formation of the aqueous humor *except* _____.
   A. beta blockers
   B. prostaglandin analogues
   C. alpha-adrenergic agonists
   D. carbonic anhydrase inhibitors

6. Which carbonic anhydrase inhibitor is administered orally? _____
   A. acetazolamide
   B. brinzolamide
   C. Trusopt
   D. Cosopt

7. Most ophthalmic drugs used for the treatment of glaucoma require contact lens wearers to wait at least _____ before reinserting their contact lenses.
   A. 5 minutes
   B. 10 minutes
   C. 15 minutes
   D. 30 minutes

8. Carbonic anhydrase inhibitors often share the suffix _____.
   A. *-prost*
   B. *-zolamide*
   C. *-olol*
   D. *-onidine*

FILL IN THE BLANK: DRUG NAMES

1. What is a **brand name** for betaxolol? _____

2. What is the **generic name** for Betagan? _____

3. What is a **brand name** for timolol maleate? _____

4. What is the **generic name** for Iopidine? _____

5. What is the **generic name** for Diamox? _____

6. What is the **brand name** for dorzolamide? _____

7. What is the **generic name** for Azopt? _____

8. What is the *generic name* for Alphagan? _____

9. What is the *generic name* for Combigan? _____

10. What is the *brand name* for dorzolamide and timolol? _____

11. What is the *generic name* for Isopto Carbachol? _____

12. What is the *brand name* for bimatoprost? _____

13. What is the *generic name* for DuoTrav PQ? _____

14. What is the *brand name* for latanoprost? _____

15. What is the *generic name* for Phospholine Iodide (United States)? _____

MATCHING

Match each drug to its pharmacological classification.

A. Alpha-adrenergic agonist
B. Cholinergic agonist
C. Prostaglandin analogue
D. Carbonic anhydrase inhibitor
E. Beta-adrenergic antagonist

1. _____ Timoptic

2. _____ Alphagan

3. _____ dorzolamide

4. _____ latanoprost

5. _____ pilocarpine

TRUE OR FALSE

1. _____ Children born with congenital glaucoma often have cloudy eyes, light sensitivity, and excessive tearing.

2. _____ The ending *-zolamide* is commonly used for carbonic anhydrase inhibitors.

3. _____ Prostaglandin analogues constrict the trabecular meshwork.

4. _____ Glaucoma is the leading cause of blindness worldwide.

5. _____ The risk for glaucoma decreases with age.

6. _____ Open-angle glaucoma is more common than angle-closure glaucoma.

7. _____ Miotics are drugs that dilate the pupil.

8. _____ Iritis is a condition associated with inflammation of the cornea.

9. _____ Conjunctivitis (pink eye) may be caused by a virus or bacteria.

CRITICAL THINKING

The following hard copy is brought to your pharmacy for filling. Identify the prescription error(s). (You already have the patient's full address on file.) There may be one error, more than one error, or no errors at all.

| Kathy Principi, MD   Date _____ |
| 1145 Broadway |
| Anytown, USA |

Pt. Name _____ Ellen Wilcox _____

Address _____

℞ Xalatan 0.005%   2.5ml
       Instill one drop

Refills _____

_____ Principi _____   _____

Substitution permitted   Dispense as written

1. Spot the error in the following prescription:

    _____

    A. Quantity missing
    B. Directions incomplete
    C. Strength missing
    D. Strength incorrect
    E. Dosage form incorrect

2. List three pairs of drug names that have look-alike or sound-alike issues with drugs used to treat glaucoma.

DRUG NAME	LOOK-ALIKE OR SOUND-ALIKE DRUG

RESEARCH ACTIVITY

1. According to World Health Organization (WHO) data, glaucoma is one of the leading causes of blindness globally, and the prevalence is rising. Check the WHO website (who.int/blindness/causes/priority/en/index7.html) to do research on glaucoma to try to explain why. Can this trend be reversed?

_____

_____

_____

_____

_____

CASE STUDY

You work at a retail store with a primarily elderly population. The pharmacists you work with have been noticing a recent increase in the number of patients requiring glaucoma treatment and you want to provide a pamphlet to patients that would explain their condition and treatment. They ask you to help create the pamphlet.

1. How would you describe open-angle and angle-closure glaucoma? Remember to use patient-friendly language to explain these conditions.

   _____

   _____

   _____

   _____

2. Write a concise one- to two-sentence description for each class of medication currently used to treat glaucoma. What are three medications that are within each of these classes?

   _____

   _____

   _____

   _____

3. What other images or information would you use in this pamphlet? Explain why you chose them.

   _____

   _____

   _____

   _____

16 Treatment of Disorders of the Ear

TERMS AND DEFINITIONS

Match each term with the correct definition below.

A. Cerumen
B. Equilibrium
C. Labyrinth
D. Ménière's disease
E. Otitis
F. Otitis externa
G. Otitis media
H. Tinnitus
I. Tympanic membrane
J. Vertigo

1. The waxlike substance secreted by modified sweat glands in the ear is called _____.

2. _____, the feeling of spinning in space, is a symptom of _____, a chronic inner ear disease associated with intermittent buildup of fluid in the inner ear.

3. _____ is inflammation of the ear canal.

4. The _____, a bony structure in the inner ear, is involved in maintaining _____, or balance.

5. Symptoms of _____ are intermittent or continuous whistling, crackling, squeaking, or ringing in the ears.

6. _____ is inflammation of the ear.

7. _____ is known as the eardrum.

8. _____ is typically caused by a viral or bacterial infection and observed clinically as inflammation of the middle ear.

MULTIPLE CHOICE

1. Select the **false** statement. _____
   A. Hearing loss can be caused by otosclerosis, autoimmune disease, or sudden sensorineural hearing loss.
   B. Otosclerosis may cause hearing loss and tinnitus.
   C. Otosclerosis is a disorder that causes destruction of bone in the ear.
   D. Otosclerosis is also called Ménière's disease.

2. Drugs that may cause tinnitus are _____.
   A. aspirin and alcohol
   B. diphenhydramine and scopolamine
   C. diazepam and triazolam
   D. methocarbamol and cyclobenzaprine

3. Which of the following conditions is *not* linked to vertigo? _____
   A. Ménière's disease
   B. Benign paroxysmal positional vertigo
   C. Gout
   D. Head trauma
   E. Infection

4. Symptoms of vertigo include all of the following except _____.
   A. dizziness
   B. nausea
   C. muscle weakness
   D. blurred vision
   E. disorientation

5. Meclizine should be used with caution in

_____.

A. patients with prostate disease
B. patients with asthma
C. lactating women
D. A, B, and C

6. Which is *not* a property of cerumen?

_____

A. Antiviral
B. Bactericidal
C. Water repellent
D. Lubricant

7. Carbamide peroxide 6.5% is the only approved agent

for _____ removal.
A. cerumen (ear wax)
B. water or fluid
C. bacteria
D. foreign material

8. What is the difference between water-clogged ears

and swimmer's ear? _____
A. Only swimmer's ear is caused by excessive fluid
in the ear.
B. Only swimmer's ear can cause an earache.
C. Only swimmer's ear produces inflammation and
infection.
D. Only swimmer's ear is treated with alcohol or
vinegar.

FILL IN THE BLANK: DRUG NAMES

1. What is the *generic name* for Serc (Canada)? _____

2. What is the *brand name* for dimenhydrinate? _____

3. What is the *generic name* for Transderm Scop (United States) and Transderm V (Canada)?

_____

4. What is the *generic name* for Auralgan? _____

5. What is the *generic name* for Auro-Dri Ear Drying Aid? _____

6. What is the *generic name* for Debrox and Murine Ear Wax Removal System? _____

MATCHING

Match the drug to its correct classification.

A. Analgesic
B. Cerumenolytic
C. Anticholinergic
D. Drying agent

1. _____ scopolamine

2. _____ antipyrine and benzocaine

3. _____ isopropyl alcohol and glycerin

4. _____ carbamide peroxide

TRUE OR FALSE

1. _____ Otitis externa is an infection of the
middle ear.

2. _____ The tympanic membrane is commonly
known as the eardrum.

3. _____ One scopolamine patch prevents motion
sickness for up to five days.

4. _____ A commonly used ending for local
anesthetics is *-caine*.

5. _____ Our perception of balance and movement
is a function of input from the eye, inner
ear, and sense receptors on the skin and
skeleton.

6. _____ When the ear is inflamed, otic solutions
that contain alcohol can cause stinging.

CRITICAL THINKING

The following hard copy is brought to your pharmacy for filling. Identify the prescription error(s). (You already have the patient's full address on file.) There may be one error, more than one error, or no errors at all.

```
Kathy Principi, MD          Date _____
1145 Broadway
Anytown, USA

Pt. Name _____ Ellen Wilber _____
Address _____
℞  Antivert 25mg      1 bottle
    2 tablets BID


Refills _____
___ Principi ___
Substitution permitted    Dispense as written
```

1. Spot the error in the following prescription:

   _____

   A. Quantity missing
   B. Directions incomplete
   C. Strength missing
   D. Strength incorrect
   E. Dosage form incorrect

2. List one pair of drug names that have look-alike or sound-alike issues with drugs used to treat vertigo.

DRUG NAME	LOOK-ALIKE OR SOUND-ALIKE DRUG

RESEARCH ACTIVITY

1. Treatment of balance disorders may involve physical therapy, diet, and lifestyle changes. What diet and lifestyle changes might be recommended?

   _____

   _____

   _____

   _____

   _____

CASE STUDY

A regular patient comes into your pharmacy to pick up a refill. As you help her at the register, she mentions that she will be going on a cruise for the first time in a month and is worried about motion sickness.

1. Provide two or three nonpharmacological recommendations that would help this patient prevent motion sickness.

   _____

   _____

   _____

   _____

2. What are three over-the-counter medications that this patient could take to prevent motion sickness? How do they work?

_____

_____

_____

_____

One month later, the patient comes into the pharmacy to thank you for your advice and to tell you about her trip. She states that she did a lot of swimming and seems to still have some fluid in her ear. She asks for your advice.

3. How would you differentiate water-clogged ear from swimmer's ear in this patient?

_____

_____

_____

_____

4. Assuming that that she has water-clogged ear, what are two over-the-counter treatments available for this patient? How do they work?

_____

_____

_____

_____

17 Treatment of Angina

TERMS AND DEFINITIONS

Match each term with the correct definition below.

A. Angina pectoris
B. Arteriosclerosis
C. Atheromas
D. Atherosclerosis
E. Coronary artery disease
F. Embolus
G. Hyperlipidemia
H. Ischemia
I. Ischemic heart disease
J. Myocardial infarction
K. Necrosis
L. Thrombus
M. Vasospasms

1. _____ is a condition that occurs when the arteries that supply blood to the heart muscle become hardened and narrowed.

2. Myocardial _____ is a deficient blood supply to the heart.

3. _____ are hardened plaques that have formed within an artery.

4. An ischemic heart disease, _____ is characterized by a severe squeezing or pressure-like thoracic pain brought on by exertion or stress.

5. _____ is the term used to describe cell death and may be caused by lack of blood and oxygen to an affected area.

6. _____ is a condition in which there is an increased concentration of cholesterol and triglycerides in the blood.

7. A stationary blood clot is called a(n) _____.

8. _____ is any condition in which heart muscle is damaged or works inefficiently because of an absence or relative deficiency of its blood supply.

9. _____ is a process in which plaques containing cholesterol, lipid material, and lipophages are formed within arteries.

10. Symptoms of angina may be caused by _____ that constrict blood vessels and reduce the flow of blood and oxygen.

11. _____ is a condition in which artery walls thicken and lose their elasticity.

12. A(n) _____ is a moving clot.

13. _____ is also referred to as a "heart attack"; it results in heart muscle tissue death and is caused by the occlusion of a coronary artery.

MULTIPLE CHOICE

1. Risk factors for angina include all of the following

   except _____.
   A. smoking
   B. a diet high in cholesterol and salt
   C. excessive alcohol consumption
   D. mild exercise
   E. obesity

2. All of the following drugs are used in the treatment of

   angina *except* _____.
   A. nitrates
   B. diuretics
   C. beta-blocking drugs
   D. calcium channel blockers

3. A woman was awakened in the middle of the night
   with severe chest pain. Her physician prescribed
   sublingual nitroglycerin. Which of the following
   adverse reactions is associated with sublingual

   nitroglycerin? _____
   A. Flushing of the skin
   B. Headache
   C. Stinging under the tongue
   D. A, B, and C

4. Which of the following is *not* considered a true type

   of angina? _____
   A. Stable angina
   B. Unstable angina
   C. Variant angina
   D. Microvascular angina
   E. None of the above

5. Patients using nitroglycerin transdermal patches

   should be advised to _____.
   A. wear the patch for 24 hours each day
   B. apply a patch at the onset of symptoms of angina
   C. rotate the sites on the skin to prevent skin
      irritation
   D. apply the patch directly over the heart

6. Which drug may be taken concurrently with

   nitroglycerin? _____
   A. Viagra
   B. Cialis
   C. Tenormin
   D. Levitra

7. Which nitrate dosage form is used only to treat acute

   angina? _____
   A. Nitroglycerin patch
   B. Isosorbide dinitrate tablets, IR
   C. Nitroglycerin injection
   D. Nitroglycerin ointment

8. Which statement about beta-adrenergic blockers is

   false? _____
   A. Beta-adrenergic blockers reduce the heart's
      demand for oxygen.
   B. Beta-adrenergic blockers decrease the frequency
      and severity of stable angina.
   C. Beta-adrenergic blockers increase the heart's
      demand for oxygen.
   D. Beta-adrenergic blockers are contraindicated in
      patients with asthma and diabetes.

9. How do calcium channel blockers help in the

   treatment of angina? _____
   A. They decrease heart rate.
   B. They decrease the strength of heart contractions.
   C. They reduce vasospasms and cause vasodilation.
   D. All of the above

FILL IN THE BLANK: DRUG NAMES

1. What is a ***brand name*** for isosorbide mononitrate? _____

2. What is the ***generic name*** for Dilatrate-SR (United States)? _____

3. What is a ***brand name*** for nitroglycerin patches? _____

4. What is a ***brand name*** for nitroglycerin SL? _____

5. What is the ***brand name*** for atenolol? _____

6. What is the ***brand name*** for amlodipine plus atorvastatin? _____

7. What is a **brand name** for propranolol? _____

8. What is the **generic name** for Corgard (United States)? _____

9. What is the **brand name** for amlodipine? _____

10. What is the **generic name** for Cardizem and Tiazac? _____

11. What is the **generic name** for Procardia (United States) and Adalat? _____

12. What is the **generic name** for Calan? _____

MATCHING

Patient education is an essential component of therapeutics. Select the best warning label to apply to the prescription vial given to patients taking the drugs listed.

A. STORE IN ORIGINAL
   CONTAINER
B. SWALLOW WHOLE; DO NOT
   CRUSH OR CHEW
C. TAKE WITH FOOD
D. HOLD SPRAY IN MOUTH AT
   LEAST 10 SECONDS BEFORE
   SWALLOWING
E. TAKE ON AN EMPTY
   STOMACH

1. _____ Isordil 10 mg

2. _____ metoprolol tartrate

3. _____ Nitrolingual

4. _____ nitroglycerin 0.4 mg SL

5. _____ Toprol XL 100 mg

MATCHING

Match the nitroglycerin dosage form with its therapeutic use.

A. Used for relief of acute anginal
   attacks
B. Used for prevention of anginal
   attacks

1. _____ nitroglycerin SL

2. _____ nitroglycerin patch

3. _____ nitroglycerin capsule

4. _____ nitroglycerin spray

5. _____ nitroglycerin ointment

MATCHING

Match each drug to its pharmacological classification.

A. Nitrate
B. Beta blocker
C. Calcium channel blocker

1. _____ Tenormin

2. _____ Imdur

3. _____ verapamil

TRUE OR FALSE

1. _____ Atherosclerosis is sometimes called "hardening of the arteries."

2. _____ Nitroglycerin should always be dispensed without a safety cap for easy access.

3. _____ Patients who experience angina will only have symptoms of tightness and pain near their heart.

4. _____ Calcium channel blockers are used in the treatment of stable, variable, and unstable angina.

5. _____ Unstable angina may occur at rest.

6. _____ When using transdermal nitrates, it is important to have a 10- to 12-hour nitrate-free period each day.

7. _____ Beta blockers are widely used in patients with angina and asthma because they treat both diseases simultaneously.

CRITICAL THINKING

The following hard copies are brought to your pharmacy for filling. Identify the prescription error(s). (You already have the patient's full address on file.) There may be one error, more than one error, or no errors at all.

Marc Cordova, MD   Date _____
1145 Broadway
Anytown, USA

Pt. Name _____ Carlton Peak _____
Address _____

℞ nitroglycerin 6.5mg cap
     i BID

Refills _____
     Cordova   _____
Substitution permitted   Dispense as written

---

1. Spot the prescription error: _____
   A. Quantity missing
   B. Strength missing
   C. Strength incorrect
   D. Directions incorrect
   E. Dosage form incorrect

Marc Cordova, MD   Date _____
1145 Broadway
Anytown, USA

Pt. Name _____ Bill Chris _____
Address _____

℞ transdermal NTG   #30
     1 q AM remove in 12 hours

Refills _____
     Cordova   _____
Substitution permitted   Dispense as written

---

2. Spot the prescription error: _____
   A. Quantity missing
   A. Strength missing
   B. Directions missing
   C. Directions incorrect
   D. Dosage form incorrect

```
  Anh Dang Tu, MD          Date _____
      1145 Broadway
      Anytown, USA
Pt. Name _____ Loan Nguyen _____
Address _____

Rx   isosorbide mononitrite 30mg tab
     i sl prn chest pain     #30


Refills _____

_____        _____ Tu _____
Substitution permitted         Dispense as written
```

3. Spot the prescription error: _____
   A. Quantity missing
   B. Strength missing
   C. Strength incorrect
   D. Directions incorrect
   E. Dosage form incorrect

4. List six pairs of drug names that have look-alike or sound-alike issues with drugs used to treat migraine headache or angina.

DRUG NAME	LOOK-ALIKE OR SOUND-ALIKE DRUG

5. Write a short paragraph describing the relationship between coronary arteries, exertional angina, and vasospastic angina.

_____

_____

_____

_____

_____

1. Hector Carvajal calls to renew his antianginal medication. He does not remember the name of the drug. Review his patient profile, and then make a list of the medications that are used in the treatment of angina. Develop a list of questions you might ask to identify the drug he is requesting.

Last name: Carvajal	First name: Hector	Gender: M
Address: 1906 E Denny Wy	City: Anytown	DOB: 4-12-49
Allergies: penicillin	Disc.:	Phone: 222-322-6789
Comment: $8/12 copay		
Insurance: PC	Plan: 05	Group:12345678
ID#: 526458904	Copay: $8.00	
Cardholder: Rivera	Jorge	Exp. date:

DATE	RX#	DRUG AND STRENGTH	SIG	QTY	MD	RF
1-1-08	72345	HCTZ 50 mg	1 QD	100	Johnson, C	2
1-1-08	72346	Slow K 8 mEq	1 BID	60	Johnson, C	3
1-2-08	79278	Nitrostat 0.4 mg	1 sl PRN	60	Johnson, C	1
2-24-08	81956	Cotrim DS	1 BID	20	Principi, K	
2-24-08	84358	Hycotuss	5 mL q6h	120	Principi, K	
3-2-08	72346	Slow K 8 mEq	1 BID	100	Johnson, C	2
3-2-08	79278	Imdur 30 mg	1 QD	60	Johnson, C	1
4-1-08	96346	enalapril 25 mg	1 BID	60	Johnson, C	2
4-7-08	102344	Nitrostat 0.4 mg	1 sl PRN	100	Johnson, C	4
4-10-08	105278	Nitro-Dur 5 cm^2/24 hours	1 QD	30	Johnson, C	1

ANTIANGINAL DRUG	DRUG IDENTIFICATION QUESTIONS
	1.
	2.
	3.

2. Hector claims that Nitro-Dur irritates him. What may be responsible for the irritation?

_____

_____

_____

_____

_____

Dylan is a new patient in your community pharmacy who was recently diagnosed with stable angina. He has started a few new medications and comes to you for help and advice. You talk to him first about lifestyle modifications. After questioning him, you discover that Dylan walks his dog twice a day for exercise and eats a large dinner every day.

1. What lifestyle modifications would you recommend to Dylan? Provide at least three specific and sustainable modifications for this patient.

_____

_____

_____

_____

2. Dylan was given metoprolol succinate as one of his new prescriptions. After reviewing his profile, you see that his asthma has been well controlled since he was a child. How would you warn Dylan about this potential drug-disease interaction?

_____

_____

_____

_____

3. Dylan was also prescribed Nitrostat, and the prescription states to "use as directed." How should Dylan take this medication? When should he take it? When should he or another person call 911?

_____

_____

_____

_____

A few months later, Dylan comes back to the pharmacy. He states that he has been taking his new medications and that his lifestyle adjustments are going well. He is at the pharmacy to fill a new prescription, Levitra, for his erectile dysfunction.

4. Would you fill this medication? Why or why not?

_____

_____

_____

_____

18 Treatment of Hypertension

TERMS AND DEFINITIONS

Match each term with the correct definition below.

A. Aldosterone
B. Angiotensin II
C. Angiotensin-converting enzyme
D. Cardiac output
E. Diastolic blood pressure
F. Diuretic
G. Hyperkalemia
H. Hypertension
I. Isolated systolic hypertension
J. Metabolic syndrome
K. Orthostatic hypotension
L. Elevated or prehypertension
M. Peripheral vascular resistance
N. Renin–aldosterone–angiotensin system
O. Systolic blood pressure

1. A potent vasoconstrictor, _____ is produced when the renin–aldosterone–angiotensin system (RAAS) is activated.

2. The_____ is defined as the volume of blood ejected from the left ventricle in 1 minute.

3. _____ is defined as resistance to the flow of blood in peripheral arterial vessels that is associated with blood vessel diameter, vessel length, and blood viscosity.

4. _____ is the measure of blood pressure when the heart is at rest.

5. _____ is a hormone that promotes sodium and fluid reabsorption.

6. The term for elevated diastolic or systolic blood pressure is

_____.

7. _____ is the measure of the pressure when the heart's ventricles are contracting.

8. A sudden drop in blood pressure that occurs when arising from lying down or sitting to standing is called _____.

9. The term for excessive serum potassium levels is _____.

10. _____ is the name of the enzyme that catalyzes the conversion of angiotensin I to angiotensin II.

11. _____ is defined as systolic blood pressure ranging between 120 and 129 mm Hg and diastolic blood pressure less than 80 mm Hg.

12. The_____ is activated when there is a drop in renal blood flow that increases blood volume, blood flow to the kidney, vasoconstriction, and blood pressure.

13. _____ is a drug that produces diuresis (urination).

104

14. _____ is the elevated systolic blood pressure only. Diastolic blood pressure is within the normal range.

15. _____ is an important risk factor of hypertension that promotes the development of atherosclerosis and cardiovascular disease.

MULTIPLE CHOICE

1. Side effects associated with metolazone include

   _____
   A. hypokalemia
   B. hypernatremia
   C. hyperglycemia
   D. A and C

2. What is guanfacine's mechanism of action?

   _____
   A. Relax smooth muscle and decrease peripheral vascular resistance
   B. Relax smooth muscle and reduce urethral resistance
   C. Inhibit the conversion of angiotensin I to angiotensin II
   D. Increase fluid loss and decrease vasoconstriction

3. Which of the following effects of calcium channel blockers is responsible for reducing blood pressure?

   _____
   A. increased force of cardiac contractions leading to increased cardiac output
   B. relaxation of blood vessels (decreased peripheral resistance)
   C. decreased renal blood flow
   D. increased heart rate

4. Patients who are taking which medication(s) should be advised to avoid salt substitutes?

   _____
   A. bisoprolol
   B. chlorthalidone
   C. spironolactone
   D. ramipril
   E. C and D

5. Stage 1 hypertension is classified as systolic blood

   pressure ranges between _____
   A. 130 to 139 mm Hg systolic and 80 to 89 mm Hg diastolic
   B. 100 to 120 mm Hg systolic and 70 to 80 mm Hg diastolic
   C. 120 to 129 mm Hg systolic and less than 80 mm Hg diastolic
   D. $\geq$140 mm Hg systolic and $\geq$90 mm Hg diastolic

6. All of the following are classifications for diuretics

   except _____
   A. thiazides
   B. loop
   C. calcium sparing
   D. potassium sparing

7. Pharmacy technicians should apply the warning label

   _____ to prescription vials containing potassium-sparing diuretics.
   A. MAY BE ADVISABLE TO EAT BANANAS OR DRINK ORANGE JUICE
   B. AVOID SALT SUBSTITUTES
   C. MAY CAUSE DROWSINESS
   D. TAKE WITH LOTS OF WATER

8. Select the **false** statement about ACE inhibitors.

   _____
   A. ACE inhibitors lower blood pressure by blocking the action of angiotensin-converting enzyme (ACE).
   B. Dry cough is a common side effect of ACE inhibitors.
   C. ACE inhibitors produce potassium loss.
   D. ACE inhibitors are contraindicated in pregnancy because they can interfere with fetal development of the kidneys.

9. Select the **false** statement about beta blockers.

   _____
   A. Beta blockers lower blood pressure by increasing heart rate.
   B. Beta blockers decrease peripheral resistance.
   C. Beta blockers used in the treatment of hypertension may be selective (β_1) or nonselective (β_1, β_2).
   D. Beta blockers should be used with caution in patients with asthma and diabetes.

10. Select the pair of angiotensin II antagonists.

    _____
    A. Coreg and Trandate
    B. Prinivil and Vasotec
    C. Inderal and Tenormin
    D. Cozaar and Diovan

FILL IN THE BLANK: DRUG NAMES

1. What is the *brand name* for hydrochlorothiazide (HCTZ)? _____

2. What is the *generic name* for Accupril? _____

3. What is the *brand name* for irbesartan? _____

4. What is the *generic name* for Tenex? _____

5. What is the *brand name* for benazepril? _____

6. What is the *generic name* for Vasotec? _____

7. What are two *brand names* for lisinopril? _____

8. What is the *generic name* for Micardis HCT? _____

9. What are two *brand names* for lisinopril plus hydrochlorothiazide? _____

10. What is the *generic name* for Cozaar? _____

11. What is the *brand name* for doxazosin? _____

12. What is the *generic name* for Hyzaar? _____

13. What is the *brand name* for valsartan plus hydrochlorothiazide? _____

MATCHING

Match each drug to its pharmacological classification.

A. thiazide diuretic
B. nonselective beta blocker
C. angiotensin II antagonist
D. selective beta blocker
E. aldosterone receptor blocker

1. _____ spironolactone 25 mg

2. _____ propranolol 10 mg

3. _____ acebutolol 200 mg

4. _____ eprosartan 600 mg

5. _____ indapamide 1.25 mg

MATCHING

Match each drug to its pharmacological classification.

A. thiazide diuretic
B. ACE inhibitor
C. angiotensin II antagonist
D. beta blocker
E. loop diuretic

1. _____ bisoprolol 10 mg

2. _____ Vasotec 2.5 mg

3. _____ furosemide 40 mg

4. _____ chlorthalidone 50 mg

5. _____ Atacand 4 mg

MATCHING

Match each drug to its pharmacological classification.

A. potassium-sparing diuretic
B. combined alpha and beta blocker
C. α_1-antagonists
D. direct renin inhibitor
E. beta blocker

1. _____ Tekturna 150 mg

2. _____ carvedilol 6.25 mg

3. _____ nadolol 40 mg

4. _____ triamterene plus HCTZ 37.5 mg/75 mg

5. _____ doxazosin 1 mg

MATCHING

Patient education is an essential component of therapeutics. Select the **best** warning label to apply to the prescription vial given to patients taking the drugs listed.

A. MAY BE ADVISABLE TO EAT BANANAS OR DRINK ORANGE JUICE
B. TAKE WITH FOOD
C. MAY CAUSE A DRY COUGH
D. DON'T CRUSH OR CHEW
E. AVOID PROLONGED EXPOSURE TO SUNLIGHT

1. _____ Inderal LA 120 mg

2. _____ amiloride plus HCTZ

3. _____ captopril 12.5 mg

4. _____ bumetanide 1 mg

5. _____ spironolactone 25 mg

MATCHING

Patient education is an essential component of therapeutics. Select the **best** warning label to apply to the prescription vial given to patients taking the drugs listed.

A. ROTATE SITE OF APPLICATION
B. AVOID PREGNANCY
C. MAY BE ADVISABLE TO EAT BANANAS OR DRINK ORANGE JUICE
D. AVOID SALT SUBSTITUTES AND POTASSIUM-RICH DIETS
E. DON'T CRUSH OR CHEW

1. _____ metoprolol SR 100 mg

2. _____ clonidine 0.1 mg patch

3. _____ ramipril 10 mg

4. _____ valsartan

5. _____ furosemide 20 mg

TRUE OR FALSE

1. _____ Complications of untreated hypertension include stroke, myocardial infarction, and kidney damage.

2. _____ It is dangerous to the mother and fetus to treat hypertension with any medication.

3. _____ Diuretics, especially loop diuretics, should not be taken at night to avoid nocturia.

4. _____ Sites for blood pressure control are the kidneys, heart, blood vessels, and lungs.

5. _____ When peripheral vascular resistance increases, blood pressure increases.

6. _____ High blood pressure is associated with obesity, excess dietary sodium intake, physical inactivity, and poor diet.

7. _____ Hydralazine is recommended for hypertensive emergencies (parenteral use) and is safe for use in pregnant women.

The following hard copies are brought to your pharmacy for filling. Identify the prescription error(s). (You already have the patient's full address on file.) There may be one error, more than one error, or no errors at all.

Anh Dang Tu, MD
1145 Broadway
Anytown, USA

Date _____

Pt. Name _____ Lili Olschefsky _____

Address _____

℞ Trandate 200mg tablet   #30
   i QID

Refills _____

_____   _____ Tu _____

Substitution permitted   Dispense as written

---

1. Spot the error in the following prescription:

   _____

   A. Quantity missing
   B. Strength missing
   C. Directions missing
   D. Directions incorrect
   E. Dosage form incorrect

Kathy Principi, MD
1145 Broadway
Anytown, USA

Date _____

Pt. Name _____ Will Jones _____

Address _____

℞ Prinizide   #30
   1-2 tablets daily

Refills _____

_____ Principi _____   _____

Substitution permitted   Dispense as written

---

2. Spot the error in the following prescription:

   _____

   A. Quantity missing
   B. Directions missing
   C. Strength missing
   D. Directions incorrect
   E. Dosage form incorrect

Kathy Principi, MD
1145 Broadway
Anytown, USA

Date _____

Pt. Name _____ Ellen Wilber _____

Address _____

℞ Capoten 50mg capsule   #60
   i BID

Refills _____

_____ Principi _____   _____

Substitution permitted   Dispense as written

---

3. Spot the error in the following prescription:

   _____

   A. Quantity missing
   B. Strength missing
   C. Directions missing
   D. Directions incorrect
   E. Dosage form incorrect

```
           Kathy Principi, MD      Date _____
              1145 Broadway
              Anytown, USA

Pt. Name _____ Preston Scott _____
Address _____

R̥   nifedipine 60mg XL    #30
       ss tab QD



Refills _____
      Principi
_____          _____
Substitution permitted    Dispense as written
```

4. Spot the error in the following prescription:

   _____

   A. Quantity missing
   B. Strength missing
   C. Directions missing
   D. Directions incorrect
   E. Dosage form incorrect

5. Give six pairs of drug names that have look-alike or sound-alike issues with drugs used to treat hypertension.

DRUG NAME	LOOK-ALIKE OR SOUND-ALIKE DRUG

6. Write a short paragraph **describing the relationship** between the kidneys and blood pressure control. List three classes of medication that have the kidney as their site of action.

   _____

   _____

   _____

   _____

   _____

RESEARCH ACTIVITY

Access the National Library of Medicine's Website (http://www.nlm.nih.gov/medlineplus/highbloodpressure.html) to answer the following questions.

1. Why is hypertension classified as a chronic disease of lifestyle?

_____

_____

_____

_____

2. What lifestyle changes are recommended?

_____

_____

_____

_____

CASE STUDY

Mary is a patient who uses your pharmacy regularly, and you know that she is recently pregnant. She comes into your pharmacy today to get her blood pressure checked. After having her sit for 5 minutes, you read her blood pressure at 146/93. You wait and check after another 5 minutes with similar results. You tell Mary that her blood pressure reading is high.

1. According to this measurement, Mary is in which stage of hypertension?

_____

_____

_____

2. Should Mary seek additional medical attention for her blood pressure? Why or why not?

_____

_____

_____

Two weeks later, Mary comes back with new prescriptions for lisinopril and hydrochlorothiazide.

3. Should the pharmacist fill both of these medications for Mary? Why or why not? (Hint: Look up the pregnancy category for these medications.)

_____

_____

_____

_____

4. What lifestyle modifications can Mary make to reduce her blood pressure? Describe at least three specific and sustainable steps she can take.

_____

_____

_____

_____

19 Treatment of Heart Disease and Stroke

TERMS AND DEFINITIONS

Match each term with the correct definition below.

A. Anticoagulant
B. Antiplatelet drug
C. Antithrombotic
D. Atherosclerosis
E. Atherothrombosis
F. Cardioglycosides
G. Cholesterol
H. Ejection fraction
I. Heart failure
J. Hemostasis
K. High-density lipoprotein (HDL)
L. Hyperlipidemia
M. Myocardial infarction
N. Ischemia
O. Low-density lipoprotein (LDL)
P. Natriuretic peptides
Q. Partial thromboplastin time (PTT)
R. Platelets
S. Plaque
T. Positive inotropic effect
U. Prothrombin time (PT)
V. Thrombolytic
W. Tissue plasminogen activator (TPA)
X. Transient ischemic attack (TIA)
Y. Triglycerides

1. A(n) _____ is a drug that prevents accumulation of platelets, thereby blocking an important step in the clot formation process.

2. _____ are metabolized to very low-density lipoproteins and are a form of energy storage found in fat tissue muscle.

3. Hormones that play a role in cardiac physiology and homeostasis are called _____.

4. _____ is a test given to determine effectiveness of heparin, while _____ is a test given to determine the effectiveness of warfarin.

5. A drug that inhibits clot formation by reducing the action of thrombin is called _____.

6. "Bad cholesterol" is known as _____, and "good cholesterol" is known as _____.

7. _____ is a condition characterized by excess fatty substances in the blood.

8. The formation of _____, or fatty cholesterol deposits, contributes to worsening atherosclerosis.

9. A(n) _____ occurs when there is a sudden loss of blood supply to a certain area, such as the heart or the brain, resulting in cell death.

10. A disease in which the heart cannot pump enough blood to meet the body's metabolic needs is known as _____ .

11. A(n) _____ is considered a stroke that lasts for only a few minutes.

12. A naturally occurring thrombolytic substance is called _____.

13. _____ are found in the blood and play an active role in the coagulation process.

14. When the force of myocardial contractions has increased, that is considered a _____ .

15. _____ is a disease characterized by the buildup of lipids and plaque inside artery walls. This buildup impedes blood flow and oxygen.

16. The heart is said to have a low _____ if it pumps only a small amount of blood from the ventricles with each heartbeat.

17. The process of stopping blood flow is called _____.

18. _____ is/are a class of medications that has the ability to alter cardiovascular function.

19. The reduction of blood supplied to tissues that is typically caused by blood vessel obstruction due to artherosclerosis, stenosis, or plaque is called _____ .

20. Excess _____ can cause atherosclerosis, but this naturally occurring substance is also needed to synthesize vitamin D.

21. A class of drugs that is used to dissolve existing blood clots is known as _____ .

22. _____ is the formation of a clot inside an artery.

23. A class of medication that is used to prevent clot formation and prolong coagulation is known as _____.

MULTIPLE CHOICE

1. Which of the following statement(s) about digoxin is/are **true**?
   A. It increases heart rate
   B. It decreases exercise tolerance
   C. It increases the force of myocardial contractions
   D. A and C

2. Regarding compensatory mechanisms that are "switched on" when the heart function fails, which of the following is **false**?
   A. The renin–aldosterone–angiotensin system (RAAS) is activated to increase blood volume.
   B. The RAAS is activated to increase cardiac output.
   C. Natriuretic peptides are released to promote vasoconstriction.
   D. Natriuretic peptides are released to promote sodium and water elimination by the kidneys.

3. All of the following drugs are used in the treatment of heart failure except_____.
   A. angiotensin II receptor antagonists
   B. "statins"
   C. vasodilators
   D. NSAIDs

4. Modifiable heart attack and stroke risk factors include _____.
   A. diet
   B. smoking
   C. alcohol consumption
   D. B and C
   E. All of the above

5. _____ typically causes hemorrhagic strokes.
   A. An embolism
   B. An aneurysm
   C. Atherosclerosis
   D. Ischemia

6. Select the class of drug that is not used in the treatment of MI or stroke. _____
   A. Anticoagulants
   B. Antiplatelets
   C. ACE inhibitors
   D. Antihyperlipidemics
   E. Thrombolytics

7. Which of the following nonprescription drugs and supplements can enhance the effect of antiplatelet medications?
   A. NSAIDs
   B. Garlic
   C. Fish oil
   D. All of the above

8. Which of the following antiplatelet drugs must be administered parenterally? _____
   A. aspirin
   B. abciximab
   C. clopidogrel
   D. dipyridamole
   E. ticlopidine

9. The antidote for warfarin overdose is

   _____ , whereas the heparin overdose

   antidote is _____
   A. vitamin D; protamine zinc
   B. vitamin D; protamine sulfate
   C. vitamin K; Digibind
   D. Digibind; vitamin K
   E. vitamin K; protamine sulfate

10. Which drug class do prescribers prefer for pregnant women with hyperlipidemia? _____
   A. Statins
   B. Bile acid sequestrants
   C. Fibric acid derivatives
   D. Nicotinic acid derivatives

FILL IN THE BLANK: DRUG NAMES

1. What is the *generic name* for Plavix? _____

2. What is the *brand name* for dipyridamole? _____

3. What is the *generic name* for Ticlid? _____

4. What is the *generic name* for Coumadin? _____

5. What is the *brand name* for dalteparin? _____

6. What is the *generic name* for Lovenox? _____

7. What is a *brand name* for heparin sodium? _____

8. What is the *generic name* for Innohep? _____

9. What is the *brand name* for alteplase? _____

10. What is the *generic name* for Lipitor? _____

11. What is the *brand name* for pravastatin? _____

12. What is the *generic name* for Crestor? _____

13. What is the *generic name* for Vytorin? _____

14. What is the *brand name* for niacin plus lovastatin? _____

15. What is the *brand name* for colestipol? _____

16. What is the *brand name* for chlorothiazide? _____

17. What is the *generic name* for Bumex (United States) and Burinex (Canada)?

_____

18. What is the *generic name* for Aldactone? _____

19. What is the *generic name* for Zebeta (United States) and Monocor (Canada)?

_____

20. What is the *brand name* for benazepril? _____

21. What is the *generic name* for Cozaar? _____

22. What is the *generic name* for Apresoline? _____

23. What is the *brand name* for isosorbide dinitrate? _____

MATCHING

Match each drug to its pharmacological classification. Each class may be used more than once.

A. thiazide diuretic
B. ACE inhibitor
C. angiotensin II antagonist
D. combined alpha and beta blocker
E. vasodilator

1. _____ carvedilol

2. _____ candesartan

3. _____ hydralazine

4. _____ indapamide

5. _____ chlorthalidone

6. _____ benazepril

MATCHING

Match each drug to its pharmacological classification. (Each class may be used more than once.)

A. antiplatelet
B. thrombolytic
C. antihyperlipidemic
D. anticoagulant

1. _____ Lovenox

2. _____ reteplase

3. _____ Livalo

4. _____ clopidogrel

5. _____ eptifibatide

6. _____ ticlopidine

7. _____ alteplase

8. _____ fondaparinux

9. _____ Lescol

10. _____ cholestyramine

11. _____ Aggrastat

12. _____ Tricor

13. _____ warfarin

14. _____ lovastatin

15. _____ aspirin

16. _____ Pradaxa

MATCHING

Patient education is an essential component of therapeutics. Select the best warning label to apply to the prescription vial given to patients taking the drugs listed.

A. AVOID PREGNANCY
B. STORE IN ORIGINAL
   CONTAINER
C. TAKE ON AN EMPTY
   STOMACH
D. AVOID ALCOHOL

1. _____ gemfibrozil

2. _____ Niaspan

3. _____ warfarin

4. _____ Pradaxa

TRUE OR FALSE

1. _____ Prothrombin time test is also known as INR test.

2. _____ Symptoms of a myocardial infarction last 1 to 5 minutes and may be relieved by rest.

3. _____ Stroke symptoms may include confusion, facial numbness, and lost balance.

4. _____ Diseases that can increase the risk for stroke and myocardial infarction include anxiety, hypotension, and stomach ulcers.

5. _____ Anticoagulants and antiplatelets can dissolve existing clots.

6. _____ All antithrombotic medications increase bleeding risk.

7. _____ Niacin can decrease VLDL synthesis and increase HDL.

8. _____ Fibric acid derivatives might cause myositis and rhabdomyolysis, two life-threatening side effects.

9. _____ There are four heart failure stages, and stage I is the most severe.

10. _____ Food can increase the absorption of digoxin.

11. _____ Heart failure can affect the left side, the right side, or both sides of the heart at the same time.

12. _____ Hydralazine reduces peripheral resistance and has been shown to indirectly increase positive inotropic effect on the heart.

CRITICAL THINKING

The following hard copies are brought to your pharmacy for filling. Identify the prescription error(s). (You already have the patient's full address on file.) There may be one error, more than one error, or no errors at all.

```
Marc Cordova, MD        Date _____
        1145 Broadway
        Anytown, USA

Pt. Name _____ Bill Carey _____
Address _____

Rx   Hydralazine 2.5mg      #60      i BID
     isosorbide dinitrate 5mg    #60      i BID


Refills _____

     Cordova
Substitution permitted      Dispense as written
```

1. Spot the error in the following prescription:

   _____

   A. Quantity missing
   B. Directions incomplete
   C. Strength missing
   D. Strength incorrect
   E. Dosage form incorrect

```
Kathy Principi, MD      Date _____
        1145 Broadway
        Anytown, USA

Pt. Name _____ Will Jones _____
Address _____

Rx   bumetanide    #30
     1 tablet daily


Refills _____

     Principi
Substitution permitted      Dispense as written
```

2. Spot the error in the following prescription:

   _____

   A. Quantity missing
   B. Directions incomplete
   C. Strength missing
   D. Strength incorrect
   E. Dosage form incorrect

```
Marc Cordova, MD        Date 5-20-08
        1145 Broadway
        Anytown, USA

Pt. Name _____ Bill Carey _____
Address _____

Rx   Plavix 75mg tablet #60
     i tablet QID daily


Refills _____

     Cordova
Substitution permitted      Dispense as written
```

3. Spot the error in the following prescription:

   _____

   A. Quantity missing
   B. Directions missing
   C. Strength missing
   D. Directions incorrect
   E. Dosage form incorrect

```
                Kathy Principi, MD        Date 5-22-08
                   1145 Broadway
                   Anytown, USA

Pt. Name _____ Ellen Wilber _____
Address _____

℞    Coumadin 5mg tab   #30    i QD
     ibuprofen 800mg tab   #30    1 TID prn


Refills _____

     Principi
_____        _____
Substitution permitted          Dispense as written
```

4. Spot the error in the following prescription:

   _____

   A. Quantity missing
   B. Strength missing
   C. Directions missing
   D. Drug interaction
   E. Dosage form incorrect

5. Mr. Cowan has recently had a myocardial infarction, and heparin is ordered. You must prepare an IV containing heparin 42,000 units in 1 L of D5NS. He is to receive 25 mL/hr. How many units of heparin will he receive per hour?

   _____

   _____

   _____

6. Mr. Cowan is discharged early, and Lovenox 40 mg SC daily is prescribed. The pharmacy stocks 300 mg/3 mL multidose vials. How many doses are in one vial?

   _____

   _____

   _____

   _____

7. You are instructed to prepare alteplase for a recently admitted stroke patient. The usual dose is 15 mg IV bolus followed by 50 mg infused over 30 minutes and then 35 mg infused over 60 minutes. Alteplase (Activase) powder for injection comes in two vial sizes—50 mg and 100 mg. The solution has an expiration date of 1 hour after the vial is reconstituted. In this case, would you use two vials of 50 mg or one vial of 100 mg? Explain your answer.

   _____

   _____

   _____

   _____

   _____

RESEARCH ACTIVITY

1. Review the patient profile below and answer the questions.

Last name: Petrosky   First name: Joe   Gender: M

Address: 1906 E Denny Wy   Anytown, USA 98122   BD: 040346

Allergies: penicillin

Comment: $8/12 copay   Disc.:   Phone: 206-322-6789

Ins: PC Plan: 05   Group#:12345678   ID#: 526458904

Copay: $8.00

Cardholder: Petrosky   Joe   Exp. date: 12-31-08

DATE	RX#	DRUG AND STRENGTH	SIG	QTY	MD	RF
1-2-08	72345	bumetanide 1 mg	1 QD	100	Johnson, C	2
2-4-08	79278	Cardizem 180 mg CD	1 QD	60	Johnson, C	1
3-1-08	81956	Cotrim DS	1 BID	20	Principi, K	
3-1-08	84358	naproxen 550 mg	1 BID	120	Principi, K	
3-2-08	72345	bumetanide 1 mg	1 QD	100	Johnson, C	1
3-4-08	79278	Cardizem 180 mg CD	1 QD	60	Johnson, C	1
3-16-08	96346	lisinopril 10 mg	1 BID	60	Johnson, C	2
3-30-08	102344	digoxin 0.25 mg	1 QD	30	Johnson, C	4
4-12-08	96346	lisinopril 10 mg	1 BID	60	Johnson, C	1
4-30-08	102344	digoxin 0.25 mg	1 QD	30	Johnson, C	4
5-4-08	105278	Rythmol 150 mg	1 Q8h	90	Johnson, C	1
5-30-08	102344	digoxin 0.25 mg	1 QD	30	Johnson, C	3

A. Joe Petrosky brings in a renewal prescription for lisinopril. Lisinopril is manufactured by two companies. Develop a list of questions you might ask to identify the manufacturer's product he previously received.

_____

_____

_____

_____

_____

B. Review Mr. Petrosky's patient profile. Make a list of the medications he takes that are used in the treatment of congestive heart failure (CHF).

_____

_____

_____

_____

C. Explain why each of these classes of medication might be used for the treatment of CHF.

_____

_____

_____

_____

_____

CASE STUDY

Victor is a 57-year-old pharmacy patient. He is in great shape with a physically demanding job, but he eats a diet high in salt and saturated fat. He binges on alcohol on the weekends, and he takes high doses of naproxen and hydrocodone/APAP for back pain. His other medical conditions include hypertension, hyperlipidemia, prediabetes, and PTSD. He used to smoke but quit 5 years ago. He refuses to take medications for his chronic conditions because he doesn't believe he needs them.

1. What lifestyle modifications should Victor use to reduce his chances of developing heart failure? Or a myocardial infarction/stroke?

_____

_____

_____

_____

2. Of the two medications Victor takes, which is of most concern as regards a heart attack or stroke? Explain your reasoning.

_____

_____

_____

_____

3. Which class of heart failure does Victor seem to be in currently? Explain your reasoning.

_____

_____

_____

_____

A few years later, Victor comes back to the pharmacy with his son. After retiring from his job, Victor gained weight; he relied on his son to push his wheelchair. Victor's son explains that his father had a heart attack 6 months ago, which put Victor into stage II heart failure. Now, the doctors say he has progressed to stage III. Victor's son hands you a prescription for digoxin.

4. Is digoxin a proper treatment option for Victor at this time? (Hint: Refer to Table 19-3 in your textbook.)

_____

_____

_____

_____

5. What other medications should Victor be taking for his class III heart failure?

_____

_____

_____

_____

20 Treatment of Arrhythmia

TERMS AND DEFINITIONS

Match each term with the correct definition below.

A. Atrial fibrillation
B. Atrial flutter
C. Automaticity
D. Depolarization
E. Ectopic
F. Electrical cardioversion
G. Refractory period
H. Repolarization
I. Supraventricular tachycardia
J. Ventricular fibrillation
K. Ventricular tachycardia

1. The _____ is the time between contractions that it takes for repolarization to occur.

2. During _____, the atria beat between 300 and 400 beats/min, and contractions are uncoordinated.

3. The period of time when the heart is recharging and preparing for

   another contraction is called _____.

4. A(n) _____ beat is a heartbeat that occurs outside of the normal pacemaker locations.

5. Persons who have a(n) _____ have a heart rate of 160 to 350 beats per min and contractions of the atrium exceed the number in the ventricles.

6. The term used to describe spontaneous contraction of heart muscle cells

   is _____.

7. _____ is the process of applying an electrical shock to the heart with a defibrillator.

8. An arrhythmia that produces heartbeats up to 600 beats/min and

   uncoordinated contractions is _____.

9. _____ occurs in a region above the ventricles and produces a heart rate up to 200 beats/min.

10. _____ causes the ventricles to beat faster than 200 beats/min.

11. _____ is the process where the heart muscle conducts an electrical impulse, causing a contraction.

MULTIPLE CHOICE

1. The process where the heart muscle conducts an electrical impulse causing a contraction is called _____.
   A. repolarization
   B. depolarization
   C. automaticity
   D. refractory period

2. Which disease requires the most immediate medical attention? _____
   A. Atrial flutter
   B. Atrial fibrillation
   C. Supraventricular tachycardia
   D. Ventricular tachycardia
   E. Ventricular fibrillation

3. Supraventricular tachycardia is an arrhythmia that originates in an area _____ the ventricles.
   A. below
   B. above
   C. within

4. Select the nonmodifiable risk factor for arrhythmia. _____
   A. Obesity
   B. Age
   C. Smoking
   D. Excessive alcohol consumption
   E. Stimulant use

5. Which of the following is *not* a disease risk factor for arrhythmia? _____
   A. Coronary heart disease (CHD) and stroke
   B. Diabetes
   C. Thyroid disease
   D. Obstructive sleep apnea
   E. Epilepsy

6. Which of the following is true about digoxin?
   A. It is a class III antiarrhythmic.
   B. It is not approved for the treatment of atrial fibrillation in the United States.
   C. It can be administered orally or IV.
   D. The therapeutic index of digoxin is high.

7. Which medication class significantly reduces first-time atrial fibrillation risk in hypertensive patients? _____
   A. ACE inhibitors
   B. Angiotensin type II receptor blockers
   C. Thiazide diuretics
   D. A and B

8. Tinnitus is a sign of _____ toxicity.
   1. amiodarone
   2. procainamide
   3. mexiletine
   4. quinidine

9. Which class I antiarrhythmic drug must be administered parenterally? _____
   A. procainamide
   B. lidocaine
   C. tocainide
   D. propafenone

10. Persons taking amiodarone may experience all of the following adverse effects *except* _____.
    A. constipation
    B. photosensitivity
    C. skin discoloration
    D. visual disturbances
    E. corneal deposits

FILL IN THE BLANK: DRUG NAMES

1. What is the *brand name* for flecainide? _____

2. What is the *generic name* for Norpace (United States) and Rythmodan (Canada)? _____

3. What is a *brand name* for propafenone? _____

4. What is the *brand name* for dofetilide? _____

5. What is the *brand name* for acebutolol? _____

6. What is the *generic name* for Corvert? _____

7. What is the *brand name* for esmolol? _____

8. What is the *generic name* for Xylocard (Canada)? _____

9. What is the *brand name* for propranolol? _____

10. What is a *brand name* for amiodarone? _____

11. What is the *generic name* for Betapace (United States)? _____

12. What is the *generic name* for Isoptin SR? _____

MATCHING

Patient education is an essential component of therapeutics. Select the **best** warning label to apply to the prescription vial given to patients taking the drugs listed.

A. DILUTE ORAL
   CONCENTRATE
B. AVOID PROLONGED
   EXPOSURE TO SUNLIGHT
C. TAKE WITH FOOD
D. TAKE ON AN EMPTY
   STOMACH
E. PROTECT FROM MOISTURE

1. _____ dofetilide

2. _____ mexiletine

3. _____ procainamide

4. _____ propranolol

5. _____ amiodarone

MATCHING

Match each drug to its pharmacological classification.

A. Class Ia
B. Ca^{2+} channel blockade
C. K^+ channel blockade
D. Class Ic
E. Class Ib

1. _____ amiodarone

2. _____ lidocaine

3. _____ flecainide

4. _____ disopyramide

5. _____ verapamil

TRUE OR FALSE

1. _____ Class I antiarrhythmic agents can produce local anesthesia.

2. _____ Beta blockers are the only drug class for the primary management of ventricular arrhythmias.

3. _____ Nonmodifiable risk factors for atrial fibrillation include age, emotional stress, gender, and bradycardia.

4. _____ Atrial flutter treatments include the antiarrhythmic medications quinidine gluconate and esmolol.

5. _____ Calcium channel blockers can cause headache, flushing, and peripheral edema.

CRITICAL THINKING

The following hard copies are brought to your pharmacy for filling. Identify the prescription error(s). (You already have the patient's full address on file.) There may be one error, more than one error, or no errors at all.

```
┌─────────────────────────────────────────────┐
│          Anh Dang Tu, MD      Date _____    │
│            1145 Broadway                      │
│            Anytown, USA                       │
│                                               │
│  Pt. Name_____Sheila Alvater_____     │
│  Address _____    │
│  ℞   disopyramide CR   #30                    │
│        1 tab BID                              │
│                                               │
│                                               │
│  Refills _____                               │
│                           AD Tu               │
│  _____    _____        │
│  Substitution permitted   Dispense as written │
└─────────────────────────────────────────────┘
```

1. Spot the error in the following prescription:

   _____

   A. Quantity missing
   B. Directions incomplete
   C. Strength missing
   D. Strength incorrect
   E. Dosage form incorrect

2. Give six pairs of drug names that have look-alike or sound-alike issues with drugs used to treat arrhythmias.

DRUG NAME	LOOK-ALIKE OR SOUND-ALIKE DRUG

RESEARCH ACTIVITY

1. Dan Cowan calls to renew his antiarrhythmic drug. He does not remember the name.
   Review his patient profile, and then make a list of the medications that are used in the treatment of arrhythmia.
   Develop a list of questions you might ask to identify the drug he is requesting.

Last name: Cowan	First name: Dan	Gender: M
Address: 1906 E Denny Wy	City: Anytown	DOB: 02-13-46
Allergies: penicillin		
Comment: $8/12 copay	Disc.:	Phone: 206-322-6789
Insurance: PC	Plan: 05	Group#: 12345678
ID#: 526458904	Copay: $8.00*	
Cardholder: Cowan	Dan	Exp. date:

DATE	RX#	DRUG AND STRENGTH	SIG	QTY	MD	RF
1-2-08	72345	furosemide 40 mg	1 QD	100	Johnson	2
1-2-08	72346	K-Dur 20 mEq	1 BID	120	Johnson	3
2-2-08	81956	Niaspan 750 mg	1 BID	100	Johnson	
2-9-08	79278	ASA gr 5	1 QD	100	Johnson	1
2-9-08	79279	Monopril 10 mg	1 QD	30	Johnson	2
3-1-08	79279	Monopril 10 mg	1 QD	60	Johnson	1
4-25-08	84639	Lescol 40 mg	1 QD	30	Johnson	1
5-2-08	102344	Betapace 160 mg	1 BID	25	Johnson	4
5-2-08	96346	Ticlid 250 mg	1 BID	60	Johnson	1
5-23-08	100013	Lipitor 10 mg	1 QD	60	Johnson	
6-4-08	105278	Norpace CR 100 mg	1 BID	60	Johnson	
7-1-08	110129	amiodarone 200 mg	1 q12h	60	Johnson	

ANTIPARKINSON DRUG	DRUG IDENTIFICATION QUESTIONS
	1.
	2.
	3.

CASE STUDY

Brady is a 63-year-old male and a regular pharmacy patient. He eats well, exercises often, and is without chronic conditions. He has never smoked, but drinks a few beers weekly. Today, he walks in with a new prescription for valsartan. Brady tells you the doctor put him on the medication for stroke prevention to keep his heart from "beating weird."

1. What condition is Brady's physician trying to prevent? How does that condition relate to having a stroke?

_____

_____

_____

2. How does valsartan help prevent this condition?

_____

_____

_____

A few months later, Brady returns with a new prescription for amiodarone. He says that he got an infection that brought him to the hospital, and the physical stress from the infection caused an arrhythmia. He asks you for advice on his new medication.

3. What class of antiarrhythmic agents is amiodarone in? How does amiodarone work to treat arrhythmias?

_____

_____

_____

_____

4. What side effects should you warn Brady of before starting this medication?

_____

_____

_____

5. You want to warn Brady that all antiarrhythmic drugs actually can cause other arrhythmias. How would you say this to Brady so that he understands the risk, yet remains compliant with the medication?

_____

_____

_____

_____

21 Treatment of Gastroesophageal Reflux Disease, Laryngopharyngeal Reflux, and Peptic Ulcer Disease

TERMS AND DEFINITIONS

Match each term with the correct definition below.

A. Duodenal ulcer
B. Gastric ulcer
C. Gastroesophageal reflux
D. Gastroesophageal reflux disease (GERD)
E. Hiatal hernia
F. Laryngopharyngeal reflux (LPR)
G. Lower esophageal sphincter
H. Peptic ulcer disease (PUD)
I. Peristalsis
J. Reflux
K. Ulcer
L. Upper esophageal sphincter

1. _____ is a motility disorder associated with impaired peristalsis.

2. The condition in which the lower esophageal sphincter shifts above the diaphragm is _____.

3. _____ is a forceful wave of contractions in the esophagus that moves food and liquids from the mouth to the stomach.

4. _____ is a condition in which stomach contents may flow upward into the esophagus to produce heartburn.

5. Backflow or _____ of gastric contents into the esophagus or laryngopharyngeal region is responsible for symptoms of PUD and GERD.

6. _____ is a term that is used to describe ulcers that are located in either the duodenum or stomach.

7. The _____ separates the esophagus and the stomach.

8. An ulcer that is located in the upper portion of the small intestine or duodenum is called a(n) _____.

9. The _____ separates the pharynx and esophagus.

10. A(n) _____ is an open wound or sore.

11. _____ is a condition in which gastric contents reflux into the larynx and pharynx.

12. A(n) _____ is an ulcer that is located in the stomach.

MULTIPLE CHOICE

1. Which of the following is *not* a lifestyle factor that worsens GERD? _____
   A. Coffee consumption
   B. Cigarette smoking
   C. Alcohol consumption
   D. Chewing gum

2. If left untreated, GERD may increase the risk for development of _____.
   A. stomach cancer
   B. asthma
   C. hemorrhage
   D. All of the above

3. All of the following may be used in the treatment of peptic ulcer disease *except* _____.
   A. cimetidine
   B. aluminum hydroxide gel
   C. sucralfate
   D. methylprednisolone
   E. lansoprazole

4. A patient taking an antacid preparation develops constipation. What combination of ingredients in antacids is likely to cause this side effect? _____
   A. magnesium hydroxide gel plus simethicone
   B. magaldrate plus simethicone
   C. aluminum hydroxide plus calcium carbonate
   D. aluminum hydroxide plus magnesium hydroxide gel

5. Chronic cough and excessive phlegm or saliva are hallmark symptoms of? _____
   A. Peptic ulcer disease
   B. Laryngopharyngeal reflux
   C. NSAID-induced ulcer
   D. Gastroesophageal reflux disease

6. Which treatment for GERD is a proton pump inhibitor? _____
   A. Tagamet
   B. Axid
   C. Pepcid
   D. Nexium

7. The No. 1 cause of peptic ulcer disease is _____.
   A. *H. pylori* infection
   B. stress
   C. drug therapy
   D. spicy foods

8. Ulcer formation is a possible adverse reaction of all of the following drugs *except* _____.
   A. aspirin
   B. lansoprazole
   C. NSAIDs
   D. prednisone

9. What is the mechanism of action of domperidone?
   A. Neutralizes stomach acid and decreases pepsin secretion
   B. Increases peristalsis by stimulating ACh release
   C. Stimulates the production of protective mucus and stomach bicarbonate
   D. Increases peristalsis by blocking peripheral dopamine receptors

10. Which drug promotes healing of ulcers and acts like a "Band-Aid"? _____
    A. cimetidine
    B. sucralfate
    C. esomeprazole
    D. misoprostol

FILL IN THE BLANK: DRUG NAMES

1. What is the **brand name** for famotidine? _____

2. What is the **generic name** for Tagamet (United States)? _____

3. What is a **brand name** for nizatidine? _____

4. What is the **generic name** for Metozolv ODT and Reglan? _____

5. What is the **generic name** for Prevacid? _____

6. What is the **generic name** for Prilosec (United States) and Losec (Canada)? _____

7. What is the **brand name** for famotidine + calcium carbonate + magnesium hydroxide?

   _____

8. What is the **generic name** for Protonix (United States) and Pantoloc (Canada)?

   _____

9. What is the **generic name** for Vimovo? _____

Chapter **21** **Treatment of Gastroesophageal Reflux Disease, Laryngopharyngeal Reflux, and Peptic Ulcer Disease**

10. What is the *generic name* for Aciphex (United States) and Pariet (Canada)? _____

11. What is the *generic name* for Reglan (United States)? _____`

12. What is the *brand name* for dexlansoprazole? _____

MATCHING

Patient education is an essential component of therapeutics. Select the **best** warning label to apply to the prescription vial given to patients taking the drugs listed.

A. TAKE 30 MINUTES BEFORE A MEAL

B. TAKE 60 MINUTES BEFORE A MEAL

C. SHAKE WELL AND DISCARD AFTER 30 DAYS

D. MAY CAUSE DROWSINESS

E. AVOID PREGNANCY

1. _____ misoprostol 100 mcg

2. _____ Prevacid 30 mg

3. _____ Pepcid 40 mg/5 mL

4. _____ metoclopramide 10 mg

5. _____ Nexium 20 mg

TRUE OR FALSE

1. _____ Ranitidine binds to both H_1 and H_2 receptors equally.

2. _____ The use of antacids such as aluminum hydroxide and calcium carbonate has fallen out of favor with better OTC options for PUD and GERD.

3. _____ Misoprostol blocks drug absorption, including H_2 receptor antagonists, proton pump inhibitors (PPIs), and some antibiotics.

4. _____ The main use of antacids is to provide a protective coating to the stomach lining.

5. _____ Stress and spicy foods can cause ulcers.

6. _____ Prescribers always combine antibiotics with gastric acid–reducing drugs to fight *H. pylori* infection.

7. _____ PPIs have the common ending *-prazole*.

CRITICAL THINKING

The following hard copies are brought to your pharmacy for filling. Identify the prescription error(s). (You already have the patient's full address on file.) There may be one error, more than one error, or no errors at all.

Anh Dang Tu, MD   Date _____
1145 Broadway
Anytown, USA
Pt. Name _____ Jon Nguyen _____
Address _____
℞ nizatidine 300mg caps once daily at bedtime
Refills _____
_AD Tu_
Substitution permitted   Dispense as written

1. Spot the error in the following prescription:

_____

A. Quantity missing

B. Directions incomplete

C. Strength missing

D. Strength incorrect

E. Dosage form incorrect

```
Anh Dang Tu, MD          Date _____
        1145 Broadway
        Anytown, USA

Pt. Name _____ Lili Ng _____
Address _____

℞   omeprazole 20mg   #30
        1/2 cap QD



Refills _____
        AD Tu
_____          _____
Substitution permitted    Dispense as written
```

2. Spot the error in the following prescription:

    _____

    A. Quantity missing
    B. Directions incomplete
    C. Strength missing
    D. Strength incorrect
    E. Dosage form incorrect

```
Anh Dang Tu, MD          Date _____
        1145 Broadway
        Anytown, USA

Pt. Name _____ Sean Price _____
Address _____

℞   Aciphex   #30
        i QD



Refills _____
        AD Tu
_____          _____
Substitution permitted    Dispense as written
```

3. Spot the error in the following prescription:

    _____

    A. Quantity missing
    B. Directions incomplete
    C. Strength missing
    D. Strength incorrect
    E. Dosage form incorrect

4. Give six pairs of drug names that have look-alike or sound-alike issues with drugs used to treat GERD, LPR, and PUD.

DRUG NAME	LOOK-ALIKE OR SOUND-ALIKE DRUG

Chapter **21 Treatment of Gastroesophageal Reflux Disease, Laryngopharyngeal Reflux, and Peptic Ulcer Disease**

5. Ms. Shorter is prescribed ranitidine 300 mg q HS. She is having difficulty swallowing the tablets and wants a liquid dosage form. Ranitidine is available 150 mg/tsp. How many milliliters must she take per dose? Please show your calculations.

_____

_____

_____

_____

RESEARCH ACTIVITY

1. Lifestyle change is an important component of treatment and prevention of ulcers. What lifestyle changes are recommended? Access the National Library of Medicine's website (http://www.nlm.nih.gov/medlineplus/pepticulcer.html) to answer the question.

_____

_____

_____

_____

CASE STUDY

Mark walks into your community pharmacy today. He is a healthy 72-year-old man with no chronic diseases. He tells you that he has been feeling increasing chest pain, especially after dinner. You gather that he gets this feeling after eating a large dinner and that the pain comes with belching and bloating. He does not smoke, but he does have a glass or two of wine a few nights weekly with dinner. When asked about the types of meals he eats, he says that he has been trying out new restaurants around town with his wife. He asks you what he can do about the pain.

1. Out of GERD, LPR, and PUD, which condition do you think he has? Why?

_____

_____

_____

2. What lifestyle risk factors does Mark have for his disease?

_____

_____

_____

_____

3. What lifestyle modifications would you have Mark implement?

_____

_____

_____

_____

4. What would be the best choice for Mark to address his symptoms: an antacid, an H_2 receptor antagonist, or a PPI? Why?

_____

_____

_____

_____

Chapter **21** **Treatment of Gastroesophageal Reflux Disease, Laryngopharyngeal Reflux, and Peptic Ulcer Disease**

TERMS AND DEFINITIONS

Match each term with the correct definition below.

A. Antidiarrheals
B. Constipation
C. Crohn's disease
D. Diarrhea
E. Gastroenteritis
F. Inflammatory bowel disease (IBD)
G. Irritable bowel syndrome (IBS)
H. Laxatives

1. _____ is an infection in the gastrointestinal (GI) tract that can cause postinfection irritable bowel syndrome.

2. Constipation is treated with _____, medicines that induce evacuation of the bowel.

3. _____ are used to reduce abnormally frequent passage of loose and watery stools.

4. _____ is a condition characterized by chronic abdominal distress, resulting in frequent diarrhea or constipation.

5. A person who has _____ has inflammation of the

   intestine, and _____ may produce inflammation anywhere along the GI tract.

6. _____ is abnormally delayed or infrequent passage of dry, hardened feces.

7. Abnormally frequent passage of loose and watery stools is known as

   _____.

MULTIPLE CHOICE

1. Which of the following gastrointestinal conditions is *not* characterized by inflammation?

   _____
   A. irritable bowel disease
   B. ulcerative colitis
   C. irritable bowel syndrome
   D. Crohn's disease

2. Select the **false** statement. _____
   A. Ulcerative colitis and Crohn's disease are inflammatory bowel diseases.
   B. Irritable bowel syndrome may be associated with abnormally low levels of the neurotransmitter norepinephrine.
   C. In ulcerative colitis and Crohn's disease, the body's immune system recognizes the bacteria that normally inhabit the GI tract as harmful invaders and releases anti–tumor necrosis factor (TNF).
   D. Ulcerative colitis produces inflammation in the upper layers of the lining of the small intestine and colon.
   E. Lifestyle modification can reduce symptoms of IBS, ulcerative colitis, and Crohn's disease.

3. Which drug(s) may be prescribed only by physicians enrolled in a drug-specific prescribing program? _____

   A. sulfasalazine
   B. alosetron
   C. tegaserod
   D. fiber supplements
   E. loperamide

4. Which of the following lifestyle modifications would help reduce symptoms for a patient with Crohn's disease? _____

   A. Limit carbonated beverages
   B. Eat small meals
   C. Reduce daily water intake
   D. A and B
   E. All of the above

5. Ulcerative colitis can affect which of the following locations? _____

   A. Colon
   B. Small intestine
   C. Mouth
   D. All of the above

6. Which statement about glucocorticosteroid use for the treatment of Crohn's disease is **false**? _____

   A. Glucocorticosteroids decrease inflammation.
   B. Glucocorticosteroids increase inflammation.
   C. Glucocorticosteroids are immunosuppressants.
   D. Glucocorticosteroids reduce flare-ups.

7. Which drug does *not* induce remission of Crohn's disease? _____

   A. azathioprine
   B. infliximab
   C. 6-mercaptopurine
   D. methotrexate
   E. olsalazine

FILL IN THE BLANK: DRUG NAMES

1. What is the *generic name* for Lotronex (United States)? _____

2. What is the *brand name* for diphenoxylate plus atropine? _____

3. What is the *generic name* for Atreza (United States)? _____

4. What is the *generic name* for Bentyl (United States) and Bentylol (Canada)? _____

5. What is the *brand name* for balsalazide? _____

6. What is the *brand name* for mesalamine (United States) and mesalazine (Canada)?

   _____

7. What is the *brand name* for natalizumab? _____

8. What is the *generic name* for Azulfidine (United States) and Salazopyrin (Canada)?

   _____

9. What is the *brand name* for olsalazine? _____

10. What is the *generic name* for Cortifoam? _____

11. What is the *generic name* for Amitiza? _____

12. What is the *brand name* for polycarbophil? _____

13. What is the *brand name* for methylprednisolone? _____

14. What is the *generic name* for Imuran? _____

15. What is the *brand name* for 6-mercaptopurine? _____

16. What is a *brand name* for infliximab? _____

MATCHING

Match each drug to its therapeutic classification.

A. serotonin receptor antagonist
B. immunosuppressant
C. immunomodulator
D. corticosteroid

1. _____ hydrocortisone enema

2. _____ alosetron 1 mg tab

3. _____ methotrexate 2.5 mg tab

4. _____ infliximab 100 mg

MATCHING

Match each drug to its therapeutic classification.

A. immunosuppressant
B. anticholinergic
C. bulk-forming laxative
D. antidiarrheal
E. aminosalicylate

1. _____ mesalamine 250 mg ER cap

2. _____ loperamide 2 mg

3. _____ Imuran 50 mg tab

4. _____ dicyclomine 20 mg tab

5. _____ Equalactin 625 mg

TRUE OR FALSE

1. _____ Crohn's disease produces inflammation and damage only in the colon.

2. _____ Ulcerative colitis and Crohn's disease are both associated with low levels of serotonin.

3. _____ One potentially serious side effect of immunomodulators is that they can reactivate dormant infections such as tuberculosis.

4. _____ Irritable bowel syndrome may be associated with abnormally low levels of the neurotransmitter serotonin.

5. _____ Toxic megacolon is a life-threatening adverse effect of alosetron.

6. _____ All commercially available aminosalicylates (5-ASA) are formulated as delayed-release products.

7. _____ Ulcerative colitis most commonly occurs between the ages of 30 and 50 years.

CRITICAL THINKING

The following hard copies are brought to your pharmacy for filling. Identify the prescription error(s). (You already have the patient's full address on file.) There may be one error, more than one error, or no errors at all.

```
┌─────────────────────────────────────────────┐
│        Anh Dang Tu, MD      Date _____     │
│          1145 Broadway                       │
│          Anytown, USA                        │
│                                              │
│  Pt. Name _____ Wilma Russell _____   │
│  Address _____    │
│  ℞   Zelnorm   #30                           │
│        i tab BID                             │
│                                              │
│                                              │
│  Refills _____                              │
│                                              │
│  _____      _____ Tu _____    │
│  Substitution permitted   Dispense as written│
└─────────────────────────────────────────────┘
```

1. Spot the error in the following prescription:

   _____

   A. Quantity missing
   B. Directions incomplete
   C. Strength missing
   D. Strength incorrect
   E. Dosage form incorrect

```
┌─────────────────────────────────────────────┐
│        Kathy Principi, MD    Date _____    │
│          1145 Broadway                       │
│          Anytown, USA                        │
│                                              │
│  Pt. Name _____ Will Jones _____   │
│  Address _____    │
│  ℞   Pentasa #28                             │
│        Insert rectally as directed           │
│                                              │
│                                              │
│  Refills _____                              │
│      Principi                                │
│  _____      _____    │
│  Substitution permitted   Dispense as written│
└─────────────────────────────────────────────┘
```

2. Spot the error in the following prescription:

   _____

   A. Quantity missing
   B. Directions incomplete
   C. Refills missing
   D. Strength incorrect
   E. Dosage form missing

RESEARCH ACTIVITY

1. How is the function of the immune system linked to ulcerative colitis and Crohn's disease? Access the website of the National Digestive Diseases Information Clearinghouse (http://www.digestive.niddk.nih.gov) to answer the question.

_____

_____

_____

_____

_____

Chapter **22** **Treatment of Irritable Bowel Syndrome, Ulcerative Colitis, and Crohn's Disease**

Lucy comes into your pharmacy today with a new prescription for lubiprostone. After asking about her new condition, she states that she has been recently diagnosed with irritable bowel syndrome. She doesn't understand how she could get the disease since she is 32 years old and in relatively good health. She is interested in hearing more about irritable bowel syndrome, as her doctor didn't explain it in great detail.

1. How would you explain her recent diagnosis of IBS? What is IBS and at what age do patients tend to see symptoms?

   _____

   _____

   _____

   _____

2. How will lubiprostone help with her IBS? What side effects can the medication have?

   _____

   _____

   _____

3. What lifestyle modifications can Lucy utilize to reduce her IBS symptoms?

   _____

   _____

   _____

   _____

After a few months, Lucy comes back to the pharmacy complaining that the lubiprostone isn't helping much. She asks for your advice.

4. What other options does Lucy have if she has predominantly diarrhea? What about if she has predominantly constipation?

   _____

   _____

   _____

   _____

23 Treatment of Asthma and Chronic Obstructive Pulmonary Disease

TERMS AND DEFINITIONS

Match each term with the correct definition below.

A. Allergic asthma
B. Asthma
C. Bronchodilator
D. Chronic obstructive pulmonary disease (COPD)
E. Forced expiratory volume
F. Metered-dose inhaler (MDI)
G. Nebulizer
H. Peak flow meter
I. Spacer
J. Spirometry

1. Two tests that measure volume of air are _____ and _____.

2. _____ is a progressive disease of the airways that produces gradual loss of pulmonary function.

3. _____ is typically defined as a chronic disease that affects the airways, producing irritation, inflammation, and difficulty breathing; however, symptoms of _____ occur upon exposure to environmental allergens.

4. Whereas corticosteroids are used in the treatment of asthma to reduce inflammation and swelling of airways, a _____ will relax tightened airway muscles.

5. A device that creates an inhalable mist out of a liquid solution is called a _____.

6. The _____ is a handheld device that is used to measure the volume of air exhaled and how fast the air is moved out.

7. A _____ is a device that delivers a specific amount of inhaled medication. A _____ can be attached to the device to facilitate drug delivery into the lungs rather than the back of the throat.

MULTIPLE CHOICE

1. Symptoms of asthma include all of the following except _____.
   A. coughing
   B. wheezing
   C. sneezing
   D. shortness of breath
   E. chest tightness

2. _____ may serve as a trigger for an asthma attack.
   A. Warm, moist air
   B. Fragrance-free products
   C. Crying or laughing
   D. All of the above

3. Treatment of COPD involves the administration of

   _____.
   A. bronchodilators
   B. glucocorticosteroids
   C. antibiotics when infections are present
   D. oxygen
   E. All of the above

4. Which of the following drugs is *not* a "reliever" medicine prescribed for the treatment of acute

   symptoms of asthma? _____
   A. albuterol (or salbutamol)
   B. levalbuterol
   C. beclomethasone
   D. terbutaline
   E. ipratropium bromide

5. Select the **false** statement. _____
   A. Long-acting β_2-agonists (LABAs) are approved monotherapy for asthma *and* COPD.
   B. Excess short-acting β_2-agonist (SABA) use indicates poor disease management in asthma patients.
   C. Glucocorticoids reduce lung inflammation; they don't help with bronchoconstriction.
   D. Xanthine derivatives similar to caffeine have multiple mechanisms of action to help manage asthma symptomology.

6. Which of the following classes of drugs is *not* a "controller" medicine, prescribed to prevent

   symptoms of asthma? _____
   A. LABAs
   B. SABAs
   C. inhaled corticosteroids
   D. leukotriene modifiers
   E. mast cell stabilizers

7. Select the **false** statement. _____
   A. Leukotriene modifiers are administered to patients with mild asthma to reduce inflammation.
   B. Leukotriene modifiers inhibit the release of proinflammatory substances.
   C. The packet of montelukast granules may be opened and premixed hours in advance for convenience.
   D. Montelukast granules may be mixed in food.

FILL IN THE BLANK: DRUG NAMES

1. What is the *generic name* for Ventolin? _____

2. What is the *generic name* for Xopenex (United States)? _____

3. What is the *generic name* for Atrovent HFA? _____

4. What is the *brand name* for ciclesonide? _____

5. What is the *brand name* for albuterol plus ipratropium bromide? _____

6. What is the *brand name* for fenoterol hydrobromide plus ipratropium bromide?

   _____

7. What is the *generic name* for Foradil? _____

8. What is the *generic name* for Serevent Diskus? _____

9. What is the *generic name* for Qvar? _____

10. What is the *brand name* for budesonide? _____

11. What is the *brand name* for fluticasone? _____

12. What is the *generic name* for Advair Diskus? _____

13. What is the **brand name** for formoterol plus budesonide? _____

14. What is the **generic name** for Singulair? _____

15. What is the **generic name** for Accolate? _____

16. What is the **generic name** for Zyflo CR (United States)? _____

17. What is a **brand name** for theophylline? _____

18. What is a **brand name** for omalizumab? _____

MATCHING

Patient education is an essential component of therapeutics. Select the **best** warning label to apply to the prescription vial given to patients taking the drugs listed.

A. TAKE ON AN EMPTY
   STOMACH
B. SWALLOW WHOLE; DON'T
   CRUSH OR CHEW
C. REFRIGERATE; DO NOT
   FREEZE
D. DO NOT SWALLOW
   CAPSULES (FOR INHALATION
   ONLY)

1. _____ omalizumab

2. _____ Spiriva inhaler

3. _____ Accolate

4. _____ zileuton

MATCHING

Match each drug to its therapeutic classification.

A. short-acting β_2-adrenergic
   agonists
B. long-acting β_2-adrenergic agonists
C. inhaled corticosteroids
D. anticholinergic
E. leukotriene modifiers

1. _____ Pulmicort

2. _____ Spiriva

3. _____ metaproterenol

4. _____ salmeterol

5. _____ zafirlukast

TRUE OR FALSE

1. _____ An MDI canister will float to the top of a jar of water when the contents are full.

2. _____ Long-acting β_2-adrenergic agonists (e.g., salmeterol) have been associated with an increased risk of severe asthma exacerbations and asthma-related death.

3. _____ A common ending for leukotriene modifiers is -*lukast*.

4. _____ A common ending for xanthine derivatives is -*phylline*.

5. _____ Solair is for mild to moderate asthma monotherapy.

6. _____ Asthma symptoms cannot be managed with lifestyle modification only.

7. _____ Asthma is the most common chronic childhood disease.

8. _____ Research shows that COPD is primarily hereditary and not affected by environmental factors.

9. _____ The use of orally inhaled corticosteroids may cause thrush (a "yeast" infection).

141

The following hard copies are brought to your pharmacy for filling. Identify the prescription error(s). (You already have the patient's full address on file.) There may be one error, more than one error, or no errors at all.

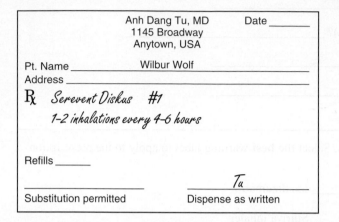

1. Spot the error in the following prescription:

   _____

   A. Quantity missing

   B. Directions incorrect

   C. Strength missing

   D. Strength incorrect

   E. Dosage form missing

2. Spot the error in the following prescription:

   _____

   A. Quantity missing

   B. Directions incomplete

   C. Strength missing

   D. Strength incorrect

   E. Dosage form missing

RESEARCH ACTIVITY

Access the National Institute of Environmental Health Sciences' website (http://www.niehs.nih.gov) and the National Heart, Lung, and Blood Institute's website (http://www.nhlbi.nih.gov/health/dci/Diseases/Asthma/) to answer the following questions.

1. The prevalence of asthma is increasing in large urban cities. What might account for this trend?

_____

_____

_____

_____

_____

2. Explain the following analogy. "The peak flow meter is to asthma management as the blood glucose monitor is to diabetes management."

_____

_____

_____

_____

_____

CASE STUDY

Carly is a patient at your retail pharmacy. She is a 27-year-old mother who has a 4-year-old son, Robert. Carly has asthma that is well controlled with Singulair plus a Ventolin inhaler for exercising. Recently she noticed Robert coughing often, especially when he's laughing and running with his preschool friends. She also noticed that his coughing gets worse when winter and spring begin. The coughing fits happen about twice a week, but Carly is concerned and asks for your advice. What signs and symptoms does Robert have? What asthma classification would you give him and why?

_____

_____

_____

_____

1. Do you think Robert's asthma is related to Carly's? Why or why not?

_____

_____

_____

_____

2. What lifestyle modifications would you recommend for Carly and her son?

_____

_____

_____

_____

One week later, Carly and Robert come back to the pharmacy with a prescription for ProAir for Robert. Carly is concerned that the doctor didn't put him on Ventolin like her.

3. What can you tell Carly about the similarities and differences between Ventolin and ProAir?

_____

_____

_____

_____

4. Considering Robert's age, would you recommend a spacer with his rescue inhaler? Why or why not?

_____

_____

_____

_____

24 Treatment of Allergies

TERMS AND DEFINITIONS

TERMS AND DEFINITIONS

Match each term with the correct definition below.

A. Allergen
B. Allergic rhinitis
C. Allergy
D. Anaphylaxis
E. Angioedema
F. Histamine
G. Immunoglobulin E
H. Leukotriene
I. Mast cells
J. Urticaria
K. Wheal

1. A(n) _____ is a hypersensitivity reaction by the immune system upon exposure to an _____.

2. Persons who have _____ experience seasonal or perennial nasal swelling and a runny nose.

3. _____ is a life-threatening allergic reaction.

4. The medical term for a raised blisterlike area on the skin caused by allergic reaction is _____.

5. An allergic response begins with the release of _____, granule-containing cells found in tissue.

6. _____ may be life threatening if swelling involves the mucous membranes and the viscera.

7. _____ is an organic nitrogen compound involved in local immune responses as well as regulating physiological function in the gut and acting as a neurotransmitter.

8. _____ is known as hives.

9. _____ is a proinflammatory mediator released as part of the allergic, inflammatory response.

10. _____ is an antibody that *is* associated with allergies.

MULTIPLE CHOICE

1. Symptoms of seasonal allergic rhinitis (SAR) include all of the following *except* _____.
   A. runny nose
   B. rash
   C. itching nose
   D. stuffy nose

2. Decongestant overuse for allergic conjunctivitis can lead to _____.
   A. rebound nasal congestion
   B. an allergic reaction
   C. rebound eye redness
   D. excessive facial angioedema

3. Which of the following is a common allergen?

_____
A. Cat dander
B. Dust
C. Mold
D. Pollen
E. All of the above

4. Pharmacy technicians are at risk for developing latex allergy. Symptoms of latex allergy include all of the

following *except* _____.
A. sneezing
B. itchy eyes
C. scratchy throat
D. hives
E. blurred vision

5. Drugs used to treat allergic symptoms include all of

the following *except* _____.
A. fexofenadine
B. Rhinocort AQ
C. cromolyn
D. pseudoephedrine
E. Nasacort

6. Cromolyn sodium _____.
A. is a leukotriene receptor antagonist
B. should begin 1 week before contact with allergens
C. is available without a prescription
D. B and C
E. All of the above

7. Steps to protect oneself from latex exposure and

allergy in the workplace include _____.
A. selecting nonlatex gloves when possible
B. using powder-free latex gloves with reduced protein content
C. avoiding oil-based hand creams and lotions when wearing latex gloves
D. washing hands with a mild soap and drying thoroughly after removing latex gloves
E. All of the above

FILL IN THE BLANK: DRUG NAMES

1. What are **brand names** for desloratadine? _____

2. What is the **generic name** for Allegra? _____

3. What is the **brand name** for fluticasone furoate? _____

4. What is the **generic name** for Xyzal? _____

5. What is a **brand name** for clemastine? _____

6. What is the **generic name** for Flonase? _____

7. What is the **generic name** for Nasacort AQ? _____

8. What is the **brand name** for cromolyn sodium? _____

MATCHING

Patient education is an essential component of therapeutics. Select the **best** warning label to apply to the prescription vial given to patients taking the drugs listed.

A. SWALLOW WHOLE; DON'T CRUSH OR CHEW
B. PROTECT FROM MOISTURE
C. SHAKE WELL
D. MAY CAUSE DROWSINESS

1. _____ diphenhydramine

2. _____ Allegra 24 hour

3. _____ loratadine disintegrating tabs

4. _____ Flonase

MATCHING

Match each drug to its therapeutic classification.

A. antihistamine
B. mast cell stabilizer
C. glucocorticosteroid
D. H$_1$ antagonist

1. _____ cromolyn sodium

2. _____ beclomethasone

3. _____ desloratadine

4. _____ Astelin

TRUE OR FALSE

1. _____ The immune system treats the allergen as an invader and produces antibodies to the substance.

2. _____ The production of allergen-specific IgE antibodies and T-cell responses directed against allergens develop after age 7 years.

3. _____ Antihistamines are not for children under 10.

4. _____ Pharmacy technicians are at risk for developing latex allergy.

5. _____ Exposure to pets early in life may reduce asthma and allergy risk.

6. _____ The use of intranasal corticosteroids may cause nosebleeds and a sore throat.

7. _____ Diphenhydramine is used to treat allergy symptoms and insomnia.

CRITICAL THINKING

The following hard copies are brought to your pharmacy for filling. Identify the prescription error(s). (You already have the patient's full address on file.) There may be one error, more than one error, or no errors at all.

```
        Anh Dang Tu, MD        Date _____
           1145 Broadway
           Anytown, USA

Pt. Name _____ Wilbur Wolf _____
Address _____

℞   Rhinocort Aqua inhaler   #1
      1-2 spray each nostril 2-3 times a day


Refills _____

_____        ____ Tu _____
Substitution permitted       Dispense as written
```

1. Spot the error in the following prescription:

_____

A. Quantity missing
B. Directions incorrect
C. Strength missing
D. Strength incorrect
E. Dosage form missing

```
                 Kathy Principi, MD        Date _____
                    1145 Broadway
                    Anytown, USA

Pt. Name _____ Will Jones _____
Address _____

R   desloratadine syrup 0.5mg/ml
     1-2 teaspoonfuls daily



Refills _____

_____Principi_____

_____      _____
Substitution permitted        Dispense as written
```

2. Spot the error in the following prescription:

   _____

   A. Quantity missing
   B. Directions incomplete
   C. Strength missing
   D. Strength incorrect
   E. Dosage form missing

RESEARCH ACTIVITY

1. What is the link between allergies and air pollution? Access the National Institute of Allergy and Infectious Diseases' website (http://www.niaid.nih.gov) and other websites to answer the question.

   _____

   _____

   _____

   _____

   _____

2. When necessary, it is possible to eliminate some allergic reactions to medications through desensitization. A common medication class used for desensitization is the penicillins. In what situations would a patient need penicillin desensitization? What is the desensitization process? Use the Centers for Disease Control and Prevention (CDC) website (https://www.cdc.gov/std/treatment/2010/penicillin-allergy.htm) to help answer these questions.

   _____

   _____

   _____

   _____

   _____

   _____

CASE STUDY

You are newly hired to a hospital pharmacy. You are learning to mix common IV solutions with sterile technique. At day's end, you take off your latex gloves and notice that your hands are red and very itchy. You also notice that your breathing has become heavy despite a lack of physically strenuous activity.

1. What symptoms of a latex allergy are you experiencing?

_____

_____

_____

_____

2. Knowing that you have a latex allergy, what steps can you take to protect yourself from latex exposure at work? Provide at least four steps.

_____

_____

_____

_____

3. What common hospital products contain latex and therefore should be avoided if possible?

_____

_____

_____

_____

4. What items outside the hospital contain latex? Write down at least three examples.

_____

_____

_____

_____

25 Treatment of Thyroid Disorders

TERMS AND DEFINITIONS

Match each term with the correct definition below.

A. Graves' disease
B. Hashimoto's disease
C. Hyperthyroidism
D. Hypothyroidism
E. Thyroid-releasing factor
F. Thyroid-stimulating hormone (TSH)
G. Tetraiodothyronine (T_4)
H. Triiodothyronine (T_3)

1. A hormone released by the pituitary gland that stimulates the thyroid gland to produce and release thyroid hormones is

   _____.

2. _____ is a hormone released by the hypothalamus that stimulates the pituitary gland to release TSH.

3. Hormones released by the thyroid gland are _____

   and _____.

4. _____, a condition in which there is an excessive

   production of thyroid hormones, is also called _____.

5. _____, a condition in which there is an insufficient

   production of thyroid hormones, is also called _____.

MULTIPLE CHOICE

1. All of the following may be used in the treatment of hyperthyroidism *except* _____.
   A. methimazole
   B. levothyroxine
   C. propylthiouracil
   D. radioactive iodine

2. What warning label should be applied to a prescription for methimazole 5 mg tab?

   _____
   A. AVOID PREGNANCY
   B. AVOID FERROUS PRODUCTS OR MULTIPLE VITAMINS WITHIN 4 HOURS OF DOSE
   C. AVOID ALCOHOL
   D. SWALLOW WHOLE; DO NOT CRUSH OR CHEW
   E. AVOID PROLONGED EXPOSURE TO SUNLIGHT

3. What warning label should be applied to a prescription for levothyroxine 0.05 mg tab?

   _____
   A. AVOID PREGNANCY
   B. AVOID FERROUS PRODUCTS OR MULTIPLE VITAMINS WITHIN 4 HOURS OF DOSE
   C. AVOID ALCOHOL
   D. SWALLOW WHOLE; DO NOT CRUSH OR CHEW
   E. AVOID PROLONGED EXPOSURE TO SUNLIGHT

4. Hormones secreted by the thyroid gland are

   _____.
   A. tetraiodothyronine (T_4)
   B. triiodothyronine (T_3)
   C. calcitonin
   D. All of the above

5. Select the **false** statement. _____
   A. When thyroid antibodies are present, autoimmune thyroid disease is diagnosed.
   B. Low-dose radioactive iodine (^{131}I) is administered to measure the amount of radioactivity taken up by the thyroid gland.
   C. High-dose ^{131}I is administered to treat hyperthyroidism.
   D. Graves' disease is an autoimmune disease that causes hypothyroidism.
   E. The full effects of ^{131}I therapy are achieved after 2 to 3 months in most people.

6. Which of the following statements is true?

   _____
   A. It takes 2 to 4 weeks of propylthiouracil therapy before maximum effects are achieved.
   B. Radioactive iodine can cause a hypothyroid state in rare cases, resulting in lifelong thyroid replacement therapy.
   C. Patients with other autoimmune diseases have higher risks of developing a thyroid disease.
   D. Hashimoto's disease is an autoimmune disorder that causes hyperthyroidism.
   E. The most common treatment for hypothyroidism is T_3 replacement therapy.

FILL IN THE BLANK: DRUG NAMES

1. What is the *generic name* for Cytomel and Triostat? _____

2. What are some *brand names* for levothyroxine? _____

3. What is the *generic name* for Tapazole? _____

MATCHING

Match each drug to its pharmacological classification.

A. thioamides
B. synthetic T_3
C. synthetic T_4

1. _____ Cytomel 50 mcg

2. _____ methimazole 5 mg

3. _____ levothyroxine 0.2 mg

TRUE OR FALSE

1. _____ Hyperthyroidism and hypothyroidism are more prevalent in women than in men.

2. _____ Liothyronine (T_3) and levothyroxine (T_4) have similar onset and duration of therapy.

3. _____ Children with chronically low levels of thyroid hormones will have no negative effects on growth and development.

4. _____ Cigarette smoking increases the risk for developing thyroid-related eye disease.

5. _____ A low TSH level signals hypothyroidism.

6. _____ Free T_4 index (FT4I) or FT4 levels are high when hyperthyroidism is present.

7. _____ A serious side effect of propylthiouracil and methimazole is agranulocytosis, especially at higher doses.

CRITICAL THINKING

The following hard copy is brought to your pharmacy for filling. Identify the prescription error(s). (You already have patient's full address on file.) There may be one error, more than one error, or no errors at all.

```
┌─────────────────────────────────────────────┐
│         Anh Dang Tu, MD      Date _____   │
│         1421 Rainier S                        │
│         Anytown, USA                          │
│                                               │
│ Pt. Name _____Howard Dean_____      │
│ Address _____      │
│ ℞   Synthroid 100mg tablet   #30              │
│     1 tab daily                               │
│                                               │
│                                               │
│ Refills _____                                │
│                                               │
│ _____    ____AD Tu_____     │
│ Substitution permitted    Dispense as written │
└─────────────────────────────────────────────┘
```

1. Spot the error in the following prescription:

   _____

   A. Quantity missing
   B. Directions incomplete
   C. Strength missing
   D. Strength incorrect
   E. Dosage form missing

```
┌─────────────────────────────────────────────┐
│         Kathy Principi, MD   Date _____   │
│         1145 Broadway                         │
│         Anytown, USA                          │
│                                               │
│ Pt. Name _____Wilma Jones_____      │
│ Address _____      │
│ ℞   l-thyroxin 25mcg  #30      1 tablet daily │
│     Prenatal vitamins with Fe #100            │
│     1 tablet daily with food                  │
│ Refills _____                                │
│     Principi                                  │
│ _____    _____  │
│ Substitution permitted    Dispense as written │
└─────────────────────────────────────────────┘
```

2. Wilma Jones brings the following prescriptions to your pharmacy. Why must you consult with the pharmacist before filling the prescriptions? What concerns might the pharmacist have with the prescriptions as written?

   _____

   _____

   _____

   _____

   _____

RESEARCH ACTIVITY

1. Pharmacy technicians should attempt to dispense the same manufacturer's product each time the patient's prescription for natural and synthetic thyroid medicine is refilled. Why is this advice given?

   _____

   _____

   _____

   _____

   _____

CASE STUDY

Mark is a 58-year-old male who frequently visits your pharmacy. He has been coming into the pharmacy in full winter gear despite an outdoor temperature around 70°F. You've noticed a slower speech and swollen face and hands. The pharmacist notices as well and talks to Mark about his symptoms.

1. Do you think Mark has hypothyroidism or hyperthyroidism? Explain.

_____

_____

_____

_____

2. Your pharmacist has convinced Mark to see a physician. What tests could the physician use to confirm or deny Mark's diagnosis?

_____

_____

_____

_____

Mark returns 1 month later with a prescription for Synthroid 100 mcg. His physician diagnosed him with hypothyroidism. His doctor also suggested he purchase a multivitamin since he hasn't been eating very well lately.

3. What should you tell Mark about the combination of Synthroid and the multivitamin?

_____

_____

_____

_____

A few months later, Mark comes into the pharmacy again to request a refill of his Synthroid. He tells you that this new prescription is working great and that he has more energy than ever. You notice that Mark cannot sit still for more than a few seconds. He is talking faster than ever, and it seems that he has lost a considerable amount of weight since the last time you've seen him.

4. What do you think is the cause of Mark's restlessness and weight loss? What can be done to reduce these symptoms?

_____

_____

_____

_____

26 Treatment of Diabetes Mellitus

TERMS AND DEFINITIONS

Match each term with the correct definition below.

A. Diabetes mellitus
B. Fasting blood glucose
C. Gestational diabetes
D. Hemoglobin A_{1c}
E. Hyperglycemia
F. Hypoglycemia
G. Insulin resistance
H. Prediabetes
I. Type 1 diabetes
J. Type 2 diabetes

1. Diabetes mellitus produces _____ (elevated blood glucose levels).

2. An adverse effect to sulfonylurea drugs is _____ (decreased blood glucose levels).

3. _____ is a condition of impaired fasting glucose (IFG) and impaired glucose tolerance (IGT) in which the body consistently has high normal glucose levels.

4. _____ may be caused by the hormones of pregnancy or a shortage of insulin.

5. Whereas a person with _____ produces little or no insulin,

   _____ is a condition in which the pancreas produces a sufficient amount of insulin but insulin receptors lack sensitivity to the insulin produced.

6. A precursor to type 2 diabetes, known as _____, is a condition in which the body does not respond to insulin.

7. A(n) _____ test is taken after a person has not eaten for 8 to 12 hours.

8. _____ is a chronic condition in which the body is unable to convert food into energy.

9. The _____ blood test measures a person's average blood glucose level over a period of weeks or months.

MULTIPLE CHOICE

1. Which of the following is a symptom of hypoglycemia? _____
   A. Frequent urination
   B. Confusion and difficulty concentrating
   C. Sweating
   D. B and C
   E. All of the above

2. Select the **false** statement. _____
   A. Insulin is released by the beta cells in the islets of Langerhans.
   B. Insulin is administered only for the treatment of type 1 diabetes.
   C. Insulin lowers blood glucose levels.
   D. Insulin may be administered by IV infusion, insulin pump, subcutaneous injection, and inhalation therapy.

3. Select the **true** statement. _____
   A. Prediabetes causes impaired fasting glucose (IFG) and impaired glucose tolerance (IGT).
   B. In type 1 diabetes, the immune system attacks and destroys the beta cells in the pancreas, so insufficient amounts of insulin are produced.
   C. In type 2 diabetes, the pancreas usually produces sufficient amounts of insulin but is unable to use the insulin effectively.
   D. Gestational diabetes may be caused by the hormones of pregnancy or a shortage of insulin.
   E. All of the above are true.

4. Elevated glucose levels may be measured by

   _____.
   A. urine glucose testing
   B. blood glucose monitoring
   C. hemoglobin A_{1c} (HBA$_{1c}$) test
   D. All of the above

5. All of the following agents stimulate insulin secretion from beta cells in the pancreas *except*

   _____.
   A. meglitinides
   B. miglitol
   C. sulfonylureas

6. All of the following agents are administered orally to

   treat type 2 diabetes *except* _____.
   A. glimepiride
   B. insulin
   C. miglitol
   D. sitagliptin
   E. metformin

7. Which of the following nonpharmacological approaches is *not* recommended in patients with

   diabetes? _____
   A. Getting 150 minutes of exercise weekly
   B. Eating a diet high in low-glycemic foods
   C. Stopping smoking
   D. Consuming multiple alcoholic drinks per day

8. Which pair of insulin products would be appropriate

   for basal-bolus administration? _____
   A. Lantus and Levemir
   B. Humalog and Humulin N
   C. NovoLog and Humalog
   D. Humulin N and Lantus

9. The mechanism of action of metformin includes the

   following *except* _____.
   A. decreasing the degradation of GLP-1
   B. decreasing hepatic gluconeogenesis
   C. increasing glucose transport across cell membranes
   D. increasing peripheral glucose uptake in skeletal muscles and adipose tissue

FILL IN THE BLANK: DRUG NAMES

1. What is the **generic name** for Humalog? _____

2. What is the **brand name** for insulin glargine? _____

3. What is the **brand name** for glyburide? _____

4. What is the **generic name** for Amaryl? _____

5. What is the **generic name** for Glucophage? _____

6. What are the **brand names** for acarbose? _____

7. What is the **generic name** for Victoza? _____

8. What is the **brand name** for repaglinide? _____

9. What is the **generic name** for Actos? _____

10. What is the **generic name** for Avandia? _____

11. What is the **brand name** for metformin and sitagliptin? _____

12. What is the **generic name** for Januvia (United States)? _____

13. What is the **generic name** for Tradjenta? _____

14. What is the **brand name** for pramlintide? _____

MATCHING

Match each drug to its pharmacological classification.

A. thiazolidinediones
B. meglitinides
C. alpha glucosidase inhibitors
D. glucagon-like peptide receptor agonist
E. sulfonylureas

1. _____ Amaryl 2 mg

2. _____ acarbose 50 mg

3. _____ rosiglitazone 2 mg

4. _____ nateglinide 120 mg

5. _____ Bydureon 2 mg

MATCHING

Patient education is an essential component of therapeutics. Select the best warning label to apply to the prescription vial given to patients taking the drugs listed.

A. REFRIGERATE; DO NOT FREEZE
B. TAKE WITH THE FIRST BITE OF A MEAL
C. AVOID ALCOHOL

1. _____ pioglitazone

2. _____ acarbose

3. _____ Humalog

TRUE OR FALSE

1. _____ A common ending for thiazolidinediones is -*glitazone*.

2. _____ Extended-release dosage forms of metformin are substitutable.

3. _____ Pramlintide can be mixed with other injectables, including insulin.

4. _____ Insulin can be used to treat type 1 and type 2 diabetes mellitus, but not gestational diabetes.

5. _____ Conventional and micronized dosage forms of glyburide are not substitutable.

6. _____ Bromocriptine is a cholesterol-lowering agent FDA approved for the management of type 2 diabetes mellitus.

7. _____ Alcohol, aspirin, and decongestants can all affect blood sugar

CRITICAL THINKING

1. Complete the table and categorize insulin according to its onset and duration of action.

ULTRA RAPID	RAPID	INTERMEDIATE	LONG

2. During a serious infection, Mr. Perkins is switched to insulin therapy: Humalog 15 units QAM and Humulin N 20 units QAM. How many days will each of the 10-mL insulin bottles last? Please show your calculations.

_____

_____

_____

_____

_____

The following hard copies are brought to your pharmacy for filling. Identify the prescription error(s). (You already have the patient's full address on file.) There may be one error, more than one error, or no errors at all.

| Anh Dang Tu, MD   Date _____ |
| 1145 Broadway |
| Anytown, USA |
| Pt. Name _____ Lili Olschefsky _____ |
| Address _____ |
| ℞ pioglitazone   #30 |
| 1 tablet daily |
| |
| Refills _____ |
| _____   _____ Tu _____ |
| Substitution permitted   Dispense as written |

3. Spot the error in the following prescription:

   _____

   A. Quantity missing
   B. Directions incomplete
   C. Strength missing
   D. Strength incorrect
   E. Dosage form missing

| Kathy Principi, MD   Date _____ |
| 1145 Broadway |
| Anytown, USA |
| Pt. Name _____ Will Jones _____ |
| Address _____ |
| ℞ Amaryl 2mg |
| 4 mg once daily. May increase up to a maximum of |
| 8mg/day as directed |
| Refills _____ |
| ___ Principi ___   _____ |
| Substitution permitted   Dispense as written |

4. Spot the error in the following prescription:

   _____

   A. Quantity missing
   B. Directions incomplete
   C. Strength missing
   D. Strength incorrect
   E. Dosage form missing

Access the National Library of Medicine's website (http://www.nlm.nih.gov/medlineplus/) to answer the following questions.

1. Why might individuals with type 1 and type 2 diabetes benefit from making lifestyle changes? Identify recommended changes, and discuss the role of nutritional supplements.

_____

_____

_____

_____

2. Why might individuals with type 2 diabetes be advised to monitor their blood glucose levels daily?

_____

_____

_____

_____

CASE STUDY

Lexie is a 17-year-old female recently diagnosed with type 1 diabetes. She comes into your pharmacy with a prescription for three vials of insulin detemir. She seems extremely worried and nervous at the drop-off counter. Lexie tells you that her physician gave her a lot of information about her new disease, but she's not sure that she can properly handle it.

1. What type of insulin is insulin detemir? When is its onset of action? When should it be administered to minimize the risk of nighttime hypoglycemia?

_____

_____

_____

2. What other products does Lexie need to properly manage her insulin therapy? Does Lexie need a prescription for these products?

_____

_____

_____

_____

3. After acquiring the necessary products, the pharmacist counsels Lexie and eases her worries. At the end of their conversation, the pharmacist recommends that Lexie keep a pack of glucose tablets in her purse at all times. Why would the pharmacist tell her to do this?

_____

_____

_____

_____

27 Drugs That Affect the Reproductive System

FILL IN THE BLANK

Match each term with the correct definition below.

A. Amenorrhea
B. Atrophic vaginitis
C. Abnormal uterine bleeding
D. Dysmenorrhea
E. Endometriosis
F. Hypogonadism
G. Hysterectomy
H. Infertility
I. Menopause
J. Menorrhagia
K. Pelvic inflammatory disease
L. Polycystic ovary disease
M. Premenstrual dysphoric disorder
N. Premenstrual syndrome
O. Supraovulation
P. Toxic shock syndrome

1. _____ is excessive menstrual bleeding; the opposite is

   _____, the absence of normal menstruation.

2. The medical term for surgical removal of the uterus is

   _____.

3. _____ and _____ are related conditions that
   have symptoms such as depression, anxiety, or irritability and are linked
   to the menstrual cycle.

4. _____ is an inability to achieve pregnancy during 1 year or
   more of unprotected intercourse.

5. _____ is a condition in which functioning endometrial
   tissue is located outside the uterus. The condition may cause

   _____ (difficult or painful menstruation).

6. _____ is a condition in which there is an inadequate
   production of sex hormones.

7. The definition of _____ is the termination of menstrual
   cycles.

8. _____ is irregular or excessive uterine bleeding that results
   from either a structural problem or hormonal imbalance.

9. _____ is a rare disorder caused by certain *Staphylococcus
   aureus* strains; the disorder is seen in women using tampons.

10. _____ is the simultaneous rupture of multiple mature
    follicles.

11. Postmenopausal thinning and dryness of the vaginal epithelium related to

    decreased estrogen levels is known as _____.

12. _____ is a condition that is characterized by ovaries twice the normal size that are studded with fluid-filled cysts.

13. _____ is an infection of the uterus, fallopian tubes, and adjacent pelvic structures that is not associated with pregnancy or surgery.

MULTIPLE CHOICE

1. Which of the following is *not* an effective method of birth control? _____
   A. foam and condom
   B. diaphragm and spermicide
   C. withdrawal
   D. oral contraceptives
   E. IUD

2. The diaphragm must be inserted sometime before sexual intercourse and should remain in the vagina for _____ after a man's last ejaculation.
   A. 1 to 2 hours
   B. 3 to 4 hours
   C. 5 to 6 hours
   D. 6 to 8 hours

3. Which of the following methods of contraception can prevent sexually transmitted infections such as HIV and syphilis? _____
   A. oral contraceptives
   B. IUD
   C. diaphragm
   D. condoms

4. Emergency contraceptives (Plan B) must be taken _____ of unprotected intercourse.
   A. within 1 to 2 hours
   B. within 3 to 6 hours
   C. within 24 hours
   D. within 72 hours
   E. within 1 week

5. How do oral contraceptives help prevent pregnancies? _____.
   A. They decrease the number of sperm excreted during ejaculation.
   B. They provide a physical barrier to prevent ovulation.
   C. They kill sperm within the vagina.
   D. They inhibit FSH and LH, preventing ovulation.

6. What condition(s) is/are treated with selective serotonin reuptake inhibitors (SSRIs)? _____
   A. Atrophic vaginitis
   B. Premenstrual syndrome
   C. Premenstrual dysphoric disorder
   D. B and C
   E. All of the above

FILL IN THE BLANK: DRUG NAMES

1. What is the *brand name* for copper-releasing IUD ? _____

2. What is the *generic name* for Aviane (United States) and Min-Ovral (Canada)? _____

3. What is the *brand name* for medroxyprogesterone acetate? _____

4. What is the *generic name* for Plan B? _____

5. What is the *brand name* for cetrorelix? _____

6. What is the *generic name* for Ovidrel? _____

7. What is a *brand name* for esterified estrogen? _____

8. What is the **brand name** for conjugated estrogens + medroxyprogesterone? _____

9. What is the **generic name** for Androderm? _____

10. What is the **brand name** for goserelin? _____

11. What is the **generic name** for Synarel? _____

12. What are **brand names** for leuprolide? _____

MATCHING

Match each drug to its pharmacological family.

A. estrogen
B. selective serotonin reuptake
   inhibitor modulator (SERM)
C. gonadotropin-releasing hormone
   agonist
D. androgen agonist

1. _____ Lupron 3.75 mg

2. _____ Brisdelle 7.5 mg

3. _____ fluoxymesterone 10 mg tab

4. _____ Estrace 2 mg

MATCHING

Match each drug to its therapeutic use.

A. infertility
B. endometriosis
C. hypogonadism
D. oral contraceptive
E. hormone replacement therapy

1. _____ danazol 100 mg

2. _____ FemHRT

3. _____ clomiphene 50 mg

4. _____ Yasmin

5. _____ testosterone

TRUE OR FALSE

1. _____ A common ending of androgen agonists is -sterone.

2. _____ Testosterone patches are *not* substitutable.

3. _____ Symptoms of menopause may include hot flashes, vaginal dryness, mood swings, and decreased sexual drive.

4. _____ Vivelle and Vivelle dot patches are substitutable.

5. _____ Androgen agonists are safe, easy-to-use medications that cause only mild side effects.

CRITICAL THINKING

The following hard copies are brought to your pharmacy for filling. Identify the prescription error(s). (You already have the patient's full address on file.) There may be one error, more than one error, or no errors at all.

<table>
<tr><td>

Anh Dang Tu, MD   Date _____
1145 Broadway
Anytown, USA

Pt. Name _____ Lili Olschefsky _____

Address _____

℞   *Nuva-Ring*

     insert one ring vaginally daily

Refills _____

_____   *Tu* _____

Substitution permitted   Dispense as written

</td><td>

1. Spot the error in the following prescription:

    _____

    A. Quantity missing

    B. Directions incorrect

    C. Strength missing

    D. Strength incorrect

    E. Dosage form missing

</td></tr>
<tr><td>

Kathy Principi, MD   Date _____
1145 Broadway
Anytown, USA

Pt. Name _____ Will Jones _____

Address _____

℞   *clomiphene 50mg*   *#5*

     Take 1 tablet daily on day 5-10 of menstrual cycle

Refills _____

    Principi _____   _____

Substitution permitted   Dispense as written

</td><td>

2. Spot the error in the following prescription:

    _____

    A. Quantity missing

    B. Directions incomplete

    C. Strength missing

    D. Strength incorrect

    E. Verify prescription is written for correct patient

</td></tr>
</table>

RESEARCH ACTIVITY

1. Anabolic steroids are controlled substances to reduce abuse. Identify health problems that are linked to abuse. Access the National Library of Medicine's website (http://www.nlm.nih.gov/medlineplus/anabolicsteroids.html) to answer the question.

_____

_____

_____

_____

_____

Morgan is a 15-year-old female who walks up to your pharmacy counter with a notebook in her hands. She says that she is required to research types of birth control for both males and females as homework for her sex education class. She asks for your help in completing this project.

1. Provide at least one advantage and one disadvantage for the following types of birth control methods:

   • Abstinence

   • Condoms

   • Diaphragms

   • IUDs

   • Oral contraceptives

   • Transdermal patch

   • Vaginal ring

   _____

   _____

   _____

2. She chose to do a research paper for the class because she is concerned that she might have either PMS or something else called PMDD. Provide at least two similarities and two differences between these conditions.

   _____

   _____

   _____

   _____

28 Treatment of Prostate Disease and Erectile Dysfunction

TERMS AND DEFINITIONS

Match each term with the correct definition below.

A. Benign prostatic hyperplasia (BPH)
B. Erectile dysfunction
C. Incontinence
D. Prostate gland
E. Prostate-specific antigen (PSA)
F. Prostate-specific antigen test
G. Urinary frequency

1. _____ is defined as the persistent inability to achieve or maintain an erection sufficient for satisfactory sexual intercourse.

2. The _____ examines the blood to measure the percentage of PSA that is unbound.

3. _____ is a protein that is elevated in men who have prostate cancer, infection, or inflammation of the prostate gland and BPH.

4. BPH and infections may produce _____, the need to urinate more often than normal.

5. Prostatitis is inflammation of the _____.

6. _____ is a loss of bladder or bowel control.

7. _____ is a noncancerous growth of cells in the prostate gland.

MULTIPLE CHOICE

1. _____ is prescribed for benign prostatic hyperplasia and male pattern baldness.
   A. Finasteride
   B. Dutasteride
   C. Progesterone
   D. Testosterone

2. Adverse reactions for phosphodiesterase type 5 (PDE5) inhibitors include

   _____.
   A. sudden hearing loss
   B. nasal congestion
   C. diarrhea
   D. B and C
   E. All of the above

3. The therapeutic effects of 5α-reductase inhibitors

   may take _____ months to be achieved.
   A. 1 to 2
   B. 3 to 6
   C. 6 to 12
   D. 12 to 18

4. The pharmacist should advise males taking finasteride

   and dutasteride _____.
   A. to use barrier contraceptives such as condoms
   B. that pregnant women and women of childbearing age should avoid contact with broken or crushed tablets
   C. may decrease desire for sex
   D. may cause erectile dysfunction
   E. All of the above

5. Which factor is *not* a cause of erectile dysfunction?

_____

   A. lifestyle
   B. heredity
   C. psychological
   D. physiological
   E. neurological

6. Select the **false** statement about drugs used for the treatment of erectile dysfunction. _____

   A. Sildenafil, tadalafil, and vardenafil are classified as PDE5 inhibitors.
   B. Cialis constricts smooth muscle and decreases the blood supply to the blood vessels that control penile engorgement.
   C. Sildenafil, tadalafil, and vardenafil are contraindicated in patients taking nitroglycerin.
   D. Alprostadil must be inserted into the urethra or by intracavernosal injection.

FILL IN THE BLANK: DRUG NAMES

1. What is the **generic name** for Uroxatral (United States) and Xatral (Canada)?

   _____

2. What is the **brand name** for doxazosin? _____

3. What is the **generic name** for Jalyn? _____

4. What is the **generic name** for Rapaflo? _____

5. What is the **brand name** for dutasteride? _____

6. What is the **generic name** for Proscar? _____

7. What are **brand names** for sildenafil? _____

8. What is the **generic name** for Cialis? _____

9. What is the **generic name** for Levitra? _____

10. What are **brand names** for avanafil? _____

MATCHING

Patient education is an essential component of therapeutics. Select the **best** warning label to apply to the prescription vial given to patients taking the drugs listed.

A. DO NOT DRINK ALCOHOL TO EXCESS

B. TAKE WITH MEAL

C. AVOID CONTACT WITH PREGNANT WOMEN

D. REFRIGERATE; DON'T FREEZE

1. _____ silodosin

2. _____ Proscar

3. _____ Cialis

4. _____ alprostadil inserts

MATCHING

Match each drug to its therapeutic classification.

A. α₁-adrenergic antagonists
B. 5α-reductase inhibitors
C. phosphodiesterase-type 5 inhibitors
D. prostaglandins

1. _____ dutasteride

2. _____ tadalafil

3. _____ terazosin

4. _____ alprostadil

TRUE OR FALSE

1. _____ Saw palmetto may reduce urinary BPH symptoms, but prostate cancer must be ruled out before starting therapy.

2. _____ A high PSA level is a sign of BPH only.

3. _____ Aggressive treatment for BPH is recommended when patients are asymptomatic or symptoms do not produce much discomfort.

4. _____ A common ending for 5α-reductase inhibitors is -steride.

5. _____ 5α-reductase inhibitors commonly cause cardiovascular-related side effects that include reflex tachycardia and postural hypertension.

6. _____ A common ending for α₁-adrenergic antagonists is -zosin.

7. _____ Chronic diseases such as hyperlipidemia and depression can cause erectile dysfunction.

CRITICAL THINKING

The following hard copies are brought to your pharmacy for filling. Identify the prescription error(s). (You already have the patient's full address on file.) There may be one error, more than one error, or no errors at all.

```
        Anh Dang Tu, MD      Date _____
          1145 Broadway
          Anytown, USA

Pt. Name _____ Wilbur Wolf _____
Address _____
℞   Flomax 0.4mg tablet   #30
      1 tablet daily



Refills _____

_____        _____ Tu _____
Substitution permitted       Dispense as written
```

1. Spot the error in the following prescription:

   _____

   A. Quantity missing
   B. Directions incomplete
   C. Strength missing
   D. Strength incorrect
   E. Dosage form incorrect

```
Kathy Principi, MD          Date _____
        1145 Broadway
        Anytown, USA
Pt. Name _____ Will Jones _____
Address _____
℞  Levitra 10mg  #10
   1 tablet up to 60 minutes prior to sexual intercourse.
   May take up to 3 doses per day if desired

Refills _____
   _____ Principi _____
_____    _____
Substitution permitted       Dispense as written
```

2. Spot the error in the following prescription:

_____

A. Quantity missing

B. Directions incorrect

C. Strength missing

D. Strength incorrect

E. Dosage form missing

RESEARCH ACTIVITY

1. Write a paragraph describing lifestyle factors that contribute to erectile dysfunction. What changes should be made to improve treatment success? Access the National Library of Medicine's website (http://www.nlm.nih.gov/medlineplus/erectiledysfunction.html) to answer the question.

_____

_____

_____

_____

_____

CASE STUDY

David is a 68-year-old male who is a familiar patient at your retail pharmacy. David comes in with a new prescription for finasteride and his recent lab results. He says that he just had a digital rectal examination (DRE) and a PSA test. On this form, you also see his free PSA count. Here is the summary of the sheet:

DRE—indicates enlarged prostate

PSA—elevated, but within normal limits

Free PSA—elevated, but within normal limits

David is still confused after his tests and examination, so he asks for your help.

1. Explain to David what each of his three results means.

_____

_____

_____

_____

2. Why did the doctor prescribe finasteride and not an alpha-1 antagonist?

_____

_____

_____

_____

3. What other condition is finasteride used for? Would you tell David about it? Why or why not?

_____

_____

_____

_____

4. What potential side effects should you inform David about?

_____

_____

_____

_____

29 Treatment of Bacterial Infection

TERMS AND DEFINITIONS

Match each term with the correct definition below.

A. Antibiotic
B. Antimicrobial
C. Bactericidal
D. Bacteriostatic
E. Broad-spectrum antibiotic
F. Microbial resistance

1. Whereas antiinfective agents that are able to destroy bacteria are

   _____, antiinfective agents that are _____
   inhibit bacterial proliferation.

2. A natural substance produced by one organism that is capable of
   destroying or inhibiting the growth of bacteria is called a(n)

   _____.

3. The term used to describe the process of bacteria developing
   mechanisms to overcome the bactericidal effects of an antibiotic is

   _____.

4. A(n) _____ is a substance capable of destroying or
   inhibiting the growth of a microorganisms.

5. An antimicrobial that is capable of destroying a wide range of bacteria is

   a(n) _____.

MATCHING

A. *ceph-* or *cef-*
B. *sulf-*
C. *-thromycin*
D. *-cycline*
E. *-cillin*
F. *-floxacin*

1. A common suffix for the fluoroquinolone family of antiinfectives is

   _____

2. A common prefix for the cephalosporin family of antiinfectives is

   _____

3. A common suffix for the macrolide family of antiinfectives is

   _____

4. A common suffix for the penicillin family of antiinfectives is

   _____

5. A common prefix for the sulfonamides family of antiinfectives is

_____

6. A common suffix for the tetracycline family of antiinfectives is

_____

MULTIPLE CHOICE

1. Select the **false** statement. _____
   A. Poverty, malnutrition, and lack of clean water increase the risk for infectious disease.
   B. Poor sanitation and inadequate housing increase the risk for infectious disease.
   C. Infectious disease is no longer a leading cause of morbidity and mortality globally.
   D. Antibiotics have played a key role in improving the survival of individuals with bacterial infections.

2. Select the **false** statement about microbial resistance.

   _____
   A. It can result in new "super bugs" that are resistant to currently available antiinfective agents.
   B. It cannot be transferred to other bacteria.
   C. It can be caused by failure to complete the full course of therapy.
   D. It can be caused by inappropriate prescribing.

3. Which of the following antibiotics is a glycopeptide?

   _____
   A. isoniazid
   B. metronidazole
   C. telavancin
   D. vancomycin

4. β-Lactam antibiotics target the bacterial cell wall. All of the following drugs are β-lactam antibiotics

   except _____.
   A. penicillins
   B. erythromycin
   C. cephalosporins
   D. carbapenems
   E. monobactams

5. Some penicillins (e.g., penicillin G and ampicillin) lack stability in gastric acids, which is why most are

   administered _____.
   A. on an empty stomach
   B. with food
   C. with a full meal
   D. sublingually

6. Select the **false** statement. _____
   A. Cephalosporins may be classified as first, second, third, fourth, and fifth generation.
   B. Clarithromycin is a key ingredient in treatment regimens for peptic ulcer disease caused by the bacteria *H. pylori*.
   C. Gastrointestinal upset is a common adverse reaction that occurs with erythromycin.
   D. Sulfonamides may be used to treat AIDS-related pneumonia (*Pneumocystis carinii*).

FILL IN THE BLANK: DRUG NAMES

1. What is the **brand name** for cephalexin? _____

2. What is the **generic name** for Suprax? _____

3. What are **brand names** for linezolid? _____

4. What is the **generic name** for Levaquin? _____

5. What is the **brand name** for clarithromycin? _____

6. What is the **generic name** for Flagyl? _____

7. What is a **brand name** for minocycline? _____

8. What is the **generic name** for Vibativ? _____

9. What is a **brand name** for sulfamethoxazole + trimethoprim? _____

10. What is the **generic name** for Bactroban? _____

11. What is the **generic name** for Cleocin? _____

12. What is a **brand name** for piperacillin-tazobactam? _____

MATCHING

Match each drug to its pharmacological family.

A. tetracycline family   1. _____ tobramycin 0.3% OS
B. sulfonamide family
C. oxazolidinone family   2. _____ linezolid 2 mg/mL
D. aminoglycoside family
E. carbapenem family   3. _____ Merrem 500 mg powder

     4. _____ Minocin 100 mg cap

     5. _____ sulfadiazine cream 1%

MATCHING

Match each drug to its therapeutic use.

A. acne rosacea   1. _____ isoniazid 300 mg
B. tuberculosis
C. bacterial meningitis   2. _____ Bactroban 2% ointment
D. pseudomembranous colitis
E. impetigo   3. _____ metronidazole 1% topical gel

     4. _____ clindamycin 150 mg cap

     5. _____ chloramphenicol 1 g powder

MATCHING

Match the cephalosporin to its correct generation. Answers may be used more than once.

A. 1st generation   1. _____ cefpodoxime
B. 2nd generation
C. 3rd generation   2. _____ ceftriaxone
D. 4th generation
     3. _____ cefepime

     4. _____ cefazolin

     5. _____ cefaclor

     6. _____ cefuroxime

TRUE OR FALSE

1. _____ The warning label TAKE WITH LOTS OF WATER is applied to prescription vials for sulfonamides.

2. _____ Oral and parenteral fluoroquinolones are contraindicated in pregnant women and people older than 16 to 18 years.

3. _____ Persons who are allergic to penicillin may also be allergic to cephalosporins.

4. _____ Tetracyclines are contraindicated in pregnancy and small children because they can weaken fetal bone, retard bone growth, weaken tooth enamel, and stain teeth.

5. _____ The milligram strength of clavulanic acid is the same for all strengths and dosage forms of Augmentin (United States) and Clavulin (Canada).

6. _____ Macrolides and penicillins may decrease the effectiveness of oral contraceptives.

CRITICAL THINKING

The following hard copies are brought to your pharmacy for filling. Identify the prescription error(s). (You already have the patient's full address on file.) There may be one error, more than one error, or no errors at all.

Anh Dang Tu, MD   Date _____
1145 Broadway
Anytown, USA

Pt. Name _____ Lili Olschefsky _____
Address _____

℞ amoxicillin + clavulanic acid tablet   #30
   i TID

Refills _____

_____   _____ Tu _____
Substitution permitted   Dispense as written

---

1. Spot the error in the following prescription:

   _____

   A. Quantity missing
   B. Directions incomplete
   C. Strength missing
   D. Strength incorrect
   E. Dosage form missing

Kathy Principi, MD   Date _____
1145 Broadway
Anytown, USA

Pt. Name _____ Will Jones _____
Address _____

℞ isoniazid 300mg
   900mg/day twice weekly with pyridoxine

Refills _____

_____ Principi _____   _____
Substitution permitted   Dispense as written

---

2. Spot the error in the following prescription:

   _____

   A. Quantity missing
   B. Directions incomplete
   C. Strength missing
   D. Strength incorrect
   E. Dosage form missing

Chapter 29 Treatment of Bacterial Infection

Kathy Principi, MD   Date _____
1145 Broadway
Anytown, USA

Pt. Name _____ Ellen Wilber _____
Address _____

℞   clarithromycin 250mg
      Take 2 tablets on day 1st day; then take one tablet
      daily on days 2 thru 5.

Refills _____

_____ Principi _____

Substitution permitted   Dispense as written

Kathy Principi, MD   Date _____
1145 Broadway
Anytown, USA

Pt. Name _____ Preston Scott _____
Address _____

℞   SMX-TMP DS capsule   #30
      i tab BID

Refills _____

_____ Principi _____

Substitution permitted   Dispense as written

3. Spot the error in the following prescription:

_____

A. Quantity missing
B. Directions incomplete
C. Strength missing
D. Strength incorrect
E. Drug possibly incorrect; verify

4. Spot the error in the following prescription:

_____

A. Quantity missing
B. Directions incomplete
C. Strength missing
D. Strength incorrect
E. Dosage form incorrect

RESEARCH ACTIVITY

Access the National Library of Medicine's website (http://www.nlm.nih.gov/medlineplus/antibiotics.html) to answer the following questions.

1. What causes antimicrobial resistance?

_____

_____

_____

_____

_____

2. What role can the pharmacist and pharmacy technician play in helping patients reduce the risk of developing resistance?

_____

_____

_____

_____

_____

CASE STUDY

Jerry walks into the pharmacy with his 9-year-old daughter Lilly. You have seen them many times before, and it doesn't take long to notice that Lilly isn't feeling very well. She coughs frequently and blows her nose often. Jerry hands you a prescription for Zithromax tablets.

1. What is the normal dosing for Zithromax? Include dose, frequency, and duration.

_____

_____

_____

_____

2. What side effects might Lilly experience when taking this medicine?

_____

_____

_____

_____

3. What would you ask Lilly before filling the prescription? (Hint: Lilly is 9 years old, and the prescription is for tablets.)

_____

_____

_____

_____

4. If Lilly feels better after 2 days, should she stop taking the medication? Why or why not?

_____

_____

_____

_____

30 Treatment of Viral Infections

TERMS AND DEFINITIONS

Match each term with the correct definition below.

A. AIDS (acquired immunodeficiency syndrome)
B. Antiretroviral
C. Antiviral resistance
D. CD4 T lymphocyte
E. Cross-resistance
F. Highly active antiretroviral therapy (HAART)
G. Oncovirus
H. Virion
I. Virustatic
J. Virus

1. The infectious particles of a virus are called _____.

2. A virus may develop _____, an ability to overcome the suppressive action of an antiviral agent.

3. A(n) _____ antiviral agent is able to suppress viral proliferation.

4. _____ is a type of white blood cell that fights infection.

5. _____ is the most severe form of HIV infection.

6. A(n) _____ is an intracellular parasite that consists of a DNA and RNA core surrounded by a protein coat and sometimes an outer covering of lipoprotein.

7. A virus may develop _____, resistance to multiple drugs in a particular drug classification.

8. A(n) _____ is a medication that inhibits the replication of retroviruses.

9. _____ is a combination of three or more antiretroviral medications taken in a regimen.

10. _____ is a virus that is an etiologic agent in a cancer.

MATCHING

A. -cyclovir and -ciclovir
B. -navir
C. -mantadine
D. -amivir

1. A common ending for antivirals that inhibit viral uncoating is

_____.

2. A common ending for antivirals used for the treatment of herpes virus infections is _____.

3. A common ending for protease inhibitors is _____.

4. A common ending for neuraminidase inhibitors is _____.

MULTIPLE CHOICE

1. HIV-infected patients are diagnosed with AIDS when

   their CD4 cell count falls below _____
   or if they develop an AIDS-defining illness.
   A. 200 cells/mm^3
   B. 300 cells/mm^3
   C. 400 cells/mm^3
   D. 600 cells/mm^3

2. Highly active antiretroviral therapy (HAART) is a
   treatment regimen for the treatment of HIV/AIDS that

   consists of _____.
   A. one antiretroviral drug
   B. one or two antiretroviral drugs
   C. two or three antiretroviral drugs
   D. three or more antiretroviral drugs

3. The risk of perinatal mother-to-child transmission of
   HIV may be reduced by the administration of a dose

   of _____ to the mother during delivery
   and to the baby upon birth or zidovudine only.
   A. zidovudine + nevirapine
   B. abacavir + zidovudine
   C. tenofovir + zidovudine
   D. Sustiva + zidovudine

4. A virus that is linked to cervical cancer is

   _____.
   A. cold sores
   B. human papillomavirus (HPV)
   C. HIV
   D. herpes zoster

5. The NRTI that may be administered as monotherapy
   for the prevention of mother-to-child transmission

   (PMTCT) of HIV is _____.
   A. zidovudine
   B. ganciclovir
   C. emtricitabine
   D. Sustiva

6. Select the **false** statement. _____
   A. Antivirals are effective only against a specific
      virus.
   B. Antibiotics are effective against viral infections.
   C. Viruses continually mutate, making it difficult to
      develop a vaccine to prevent virus infection.
   D. Antivirals inhibit virus-specific steps in the
      replication cycle.

7. Which drug is *not* prescribed for the treatment of

   cytomegalovirus retinitis? _____
   A. cidofovir
   B. saquinavir
   C. foscarnet
   D. ganciclovir

8. The steps in the HIV life cycle are

   _____.
   A. binding, fusion, and uncoating
   B. reverse transcription and integration
   C. genome replication and protein synthesis
   D. protein cleavage, assembly, and virus release
   E. All of the above

9. Nevirapine is associated with fatal _____
   toxicity, and the FDA has required changes in the
   package labeling to warn of this adverse effect.
   A. kidney
   B. heart
   C. liver
   D. thyroid

FILL IN THE BLANK: DRUG NAMES

1. What is the *brand name* for peramivir? _____

2. What is the *generic name* for Flumadine (United States)? _____

3. What is the *generic name* for Tamiflu? _____

4. What is the *brand name* for zanamivir? _____

5. What is the *generic name* for Pegasys? _____

6. What is the *generic name* for PegIntron (United States)? _____

7. What is the *generic name* for Famvir? _____

8. What is the *generic name* for Foscavir (United States)? _____

9. What is the *generic name* for Denavir? _____

10. What is the *generic name* for Viroptic? _____

11. What is the *brand name* for valacyclovir? _____

12. What is the *generic name* for Virazole? _____

13. What is the *generic name* for Ziagen? _____

14. What is the *brand name* for didanosine? _____

15. What is the *generic name* for Emtriva? _____

16. What is the *brand name* for stavudine? _____

17. What is the *brand name* for emtricitabine + tenofovir DF? _____

18. What is the *generic name* for Truvada? _____

19. What is the *generic name* for Trizivir? _____

20. What is the *brand name* for delavirdine? _____

21. What is the *brand name* for lamivudine + zidovudine? _____

22. What is the *brand name* for efavirenz? _____

23. What is the *brand name* for efavirenz + emtricitabine + tenofovir? _____

24. What is the *brand name* for atazanavir? _____

25. What is the *generic name* for Prezista? _____

26. What is the *brand name* for indinavir? _____

27. What is the *generic name* for Lexiva (United States) and Telzir (Canada)? _____

28. What is the *brand name* for Viracept? _____

29. What is the *brand name* for saquinavir? _____

30. What is the *brand name* for lopinavir + ritonavir? _____

MATCHING

Match each drug to its pharmacological family.

A. inhibitor of viral uncoating
B. neuraminidase inhibitor
C. interferon
D. inhibition of DNA replication

1. _____ Valcyte

2. _____ Relenza

3. _____ Intron-A

4. _____ amantadine

MATCHING

Match each drug to its therapeutic use.

A. herpes
B. influenza
C. hepatitis C
D. respiratory syncytial virus (RSV)
E. cytomegalovirus (CMV)

1. _____ peginterferon alfa-2b

2. _____ Tamiflu

3. _____ Virazole

4. _____ Cytovene

5. _____ penciclovir

MATCHING

Match each drug to its pharmacological family. Each answer may be used more than once.

A. nucleoside and nucleotide reverse
   transcriptase inhibitors (NRTIs)
B. non-nucleoside reverse
   transcriptase inhibitors (NNRTIs)
C. protease inhibitor
D. fusion inhibitor
E. CCR5 antagonist
F. integrase inhibitor

1. _____ nevirapine

2. _____ Fuzeon

3. _____ Norvir

4. _____ lamivudine

5. _____ rilpivirine

6. _____ Zerit

7. _____ Selzentry

8. _____ saquinavir

9. _____ raltegravir

10. _____ Kaletra

TRUE/FALSE

1. _____ Cross-resistance to similar antiviral
medications can occur, such as with
lamivudine and emtricitabine.

2. _____ Neuraminidase inhibitors are not
effective against influenza B.

3. _____ In combination with other agents,
ribavirin can treat hepatitis C. Alone it
can be used for RSV.

4. _____ HAART requires strict adherence to
every medication for a patient's lifetime.

The following hard copies are brought to your pharmacy for filling. Identify the prescription error(s). (You already have the patient's full address on file.) There may be one error, more than one error, or no errors at all.

```
┌─────────────────────────────────────────┐
│       Kathy Principi, MD    Date 1-28-05 │
│          1145 Broadway                    │
│          Anytown, USA                     │
│                                           │
│  Pt. Name _____ Ellen Wilber _____  │
│  Address _____ │
│  ℞    Videx oral solution 10mg/ml         │
│       12ml BID                            │
│                                           │
│                                           │
│  Refills _____                           │
│  ____ Principi ____    _____    │
│  Substitution permitted  Dispense as written │
└─────────────────────────────────────────┘
```

1. Spot the error in the following prescription:

    _____

    A. Quantity missing
    B. Directions incomplete
    C. Strength missing
    D. Strength incorrect
    E. Dosage form incorrect

```
┌─────────────────────────────────────────┐
│       Kathy Principi, MD    Date 1-28-05 │
│          1145 Broadway                    │
│          Anytown, USA                     │
│                                           │
│  Pt. Name _____ Ellen Wilber _____  │
│  Address _____ │
│  ℞    Tamiflu 12mg/ml    25ml             │
│       BID x 5 days                        │
│                                           │
│                                           │
│  Refills _____                           │
│  ____ Principi ____                        │
│  Substitution permitted  Dispense as written │
└─────────────────────────────────────────┘
```

2. Spot the error in the following prescription:

    _____

    A. Quantity missing
    B. Directions incomplete
    C. Strength missing
    D. Strength incorrect
    E. Dosage form incorrect

3. Give four pairs of drug names that have look-alike or sound-alike issues with drugs used for the treatment of viral infections.

DRUG NAME	LOOK-ALIKE OR SOUND-ALIKE DRUG

RESEARCH ACTIVITY

Access the *Merck Manuals* website (http://www.merck.com/mmpe/sec14/ch188/ch188d.html#sec14-ch188-ch188d-2325), the Centers for Disease Control and Prevention's website (http://www.cdc.gov), and other websites to complete the research activity.

1. What is a flu pandemic, and what is its cause?

_____

_____

_____

_____

2. How do scientists determine which strain(s) of flu to create a vaccine for?

_____

_____

_____

_____

CASE STUDY

Henry comes to your pharmacy with a new prescription. He says, "My doctor gave me this prescription for Valtrex for my genital herpes." He has a few questions about this new medication. He asks you these questions.

1. "How does this medication work to treat my condition?"

_____

_____

_____

_____

2. "What are the side effects from taking this medication?"

_____

_____

_____

_____

_____

3. "What can I do to limit the chance of spreading this to my significant other?" (Hint: Use the Internet to find more information about this topic. Suggested website: https://www.cdc.gov/std/herpes/stdfact-herpes.htm.)

_____

_____

_____

_____

As Henry leaves, another customer tells you she overheard your conversation with Henry. She's confused because she takes the same medication (Valtrex), but her doctor said to take it for cold sores. She asks you, "Did my doctor lie to me? Do I actually have genital herpes?"

4. What would you say to this patient to help ease her fears?

_____

_____

_____

5. Assuming the same dose, would Valtrex have the same side effects in Jane as in Henry? Why or why not?

_____

_____

_____

31 Treatment of Cancers

TERMS AND DEFINITIONS

Match each term with the correct definition below.

A. Benign
B. Cancer
C. Chemotherapy
D. Complementary and alternative medicine (CAM)
E. Malignant
F. Mammogram
G. Melanoma
H. Metastasis
I. Neoplasm
J. Oncovirus
K. Polyp
L. Prostate-specific antigen (PSA) test
M. Radiation therapy
N. Stage
O. Stem cell
P. Tumor marker

1. A tumor that is not cancerous is _____ and does not spread to surrounding tissues or other parts of the body.

2. _____ is a type of cell from which other types of cells can form.

3. A(n) _____ is a screening examination to detect breast cancer.

4. The spread of cancer from one part of the body to another is called _____ .

5. _____ is the extent of a cancer within the body. Staging is based on the size of the tumor, whether lymph nodes contain cancer, and whether the disease has spread from the original site to other parts of the body.

6. _____ is a test that measures level of free PSA, a protein produced by the prostate gland. Levels are elevated in men who have prostate cancer, infection, or inflammation of the prostate gland and benign prostatic hyperplasia (BPH).

7. Cancerous tumors that can invade and destroy nearby tissue and spread to other parts of the body are considered to be _____ .

8. Treatment with drugs that kill cancer is known as _____ .

9. _____ is a term for diseases in which abnormal cells divide without control.

10. _____ is a virus that is an etiologic agent in a cancer.

11. Treatments that may include dietary supplements, herbal preparations, acupuncture, massage, magnet therapy, spiritual healing, and meditation are known as _____ .

12. _____ is a growth that protrudes from a mucous membrane.

13. A substance sometimes found in the blood, other body fluids, or tissues that may signal the presence of a certain type of cancer is known as a _____ .

14. _____ uses high-energy radiation from x-rays, gamma rays, neutrons, and other sources to kill cancer cells and shrink tumors.

15. _____ is a form of skin cancer that arises in melanocytes, the cells that produce pigment.

16. _____ is another word for tumor.

MULTIPLE CHOICE

1. Which of the following is a test to screen for colorectal cancer? _____
   A. PSA
   B. Pap
   C. fetal occult blood test (FOBT)
   D. mammogram

2. Which of the following cancers is *not* linked to increased risk due to family history?
   _____
   A. breast
   B. stomach
   C. colon
   D. skin

3. Cancers are categorized by stage. Staging is based on all of the following *except* _____
   A. size of the tumor
   B. lymph node involvement
   C. metastasis
   D. length of time cancer has been present

4. Which source of ionizing radiation is *not* used for treatment of cancers?
   A. x-rays
   B. gamma rays
   C. neutrons
   D. UV light

5. A cancer that arises in the cells that produce pigment in the skin is called _____ .
   A. melanoma
   B. lymphoma
   C. leukemia

6. Which treatment would *not* be classified as complementary and alternative medicine (CAM)?
   _____
   A. dietary supplements and herbal preparations
   B. acupuncture and massage
   C. magnet therapy
   D. chemotherapy
   E. spiritual healing and meditation

7. A warning label that is commonly affixed to most prescriptions for orally administered chemotherapeutic agents for women is
   _____ .
   A. AVOID PREGNANCY
   B. TAKE WITH LOTS OF WATER
   C. SHAKE WELL
   D. AVOID PROLONGED SUNLIGHT

8. Select the **false** statement about lung cancer.
   _____
   A. Lung cancer is the most common form of cancer.
   B. A history of smoking tobacco is nearly always the cause of small cell lung cancer.
   C. Lung cancer is classified as small cell lung cancer and non–small cell lung cancer.
   D. Antineoplastic agents used to treat lung cancer are effective against both forms of the disease.

9. Which drug is *not* approved for the treatment of breast cancer? _____
   A. tamoxifen
   B. hydroxyurea
   C. Taxol
   D. Femara

10. Which of the following is *not* a common side effect of methotrexate? _____
    A. Increased appetite
    B. Hair loss
    C. Nausea
    D. Increased risk of infection

1. What is the *brand name* for fulvestrant? _____

2. What is the *generic name* for Soltamox (United States) and Nolvadex-D (Canada)?

   _____

3. What is a *brand name* for exemestane? _____

4. What is the *generic name* for Fareston (United States)? _____

5. What is the *generic name* for Arimidex? _____

6. What is the *generic name* for Femara? _____

7. What is the *brand name* for goserelin? _____

8. What is the *generic name* for Megace? _____

9. What is the *generic name* for Cytoxan? _____

10. What is the *generic name* for Taxotere? _____

11. What is the *generic name* for Taxol? _____

12. What is the *brand name* for vinorelbine? _____

13. What is the *generic name* for Adriamycin? _____

14. What is the *generic name* for Ellence (United States) and Pharmorubicin PFS (Canada)?

    _____

15. What is the *brand name* for everolimus? _____

16. What is the *generic name* for Camptosar? _____

17. What is the *brand name* for erlotinib? _____

18. What is the *generic name* for Eloxatin? _____

19. What is the *generic name* for Xeloda? _____

20. What is the *generic name* for Keytruda? _____

21. What is the *brand name* for fludarabine? _____

22. What is the *brand name* for bevacizumab? _____

23. What is the *generic name* for Gemzar? _____

24. What is the *brand name* for pemetrexed? _____

25. What is the *generic name* for Purinethol? _____

26. What is the *generic name* for Emcyt? _____

27. What is the *generic name* for Cosmegen? _____

28. What is the *generic name* for Tykerb? _____

MATCHING

Match each drug to its pharmacological classification.

A. aromatase inhibitors

B. taxanes

C. anthracyclines

D. topoisomerase inhibitors

E. vinca alkaloid

F. microtubule inhibitor

1. _____ vincristine

2. _____ teniposide

3. _____ anastrozole

4. _____ paclitaxel

5. _____ doxorubicin

6. _____ eribulin

MATCHING

Match each drug to its pharmacological classification.

A. aromatase inhibitors

B. taxanes

C. anthracyclines

D. topoisomerase inhibitors

E. platinum compounds

F. kinase inhibitors

1. _____ *-poside* and *-tecan*

2. _____ *-trozole*

3. _____ *-platin*

4. _____ *-rubicin*

5. _____ *-taxel*

6. _____ *-tinib*

TRUE OR FALSE

1. _____ Melanoma is the most treatable form of skin cancer.

2. _____ Cancerous tumors are benign.

3. _____ Specific cancers are named according to the site where the cancerous growth begins and the type of cells involved.

4. _____ A woman who has never been pregnant is at a decreased risk of breast cancer.

5. _____ Radon is a radioactive gas that if inhaled in sufficient quantity can lead to lung cancer.

6. _____ A polyp is a growth that forms on the torso.

7. _____ A lymphoma is a cancer that begins in cells of the skin.

8. _____ Metastasis is the spread of cancer from one part of the body to another.

9. _____ Implant radiation is also known as brachytherapy.

10. _____ Selective estrogen receptor modulators (SERMs) are indicated only for use in postmenopausal women.

11. _____ Doxorubicin and doxorubicin liposomal are not substitutable.

12. _____ Kinase inhibitors block signaling pathways required for tumor growth.

CRITICAL THINKING

The following hard copies are brought to your pharmacy for filling. Identify the prescription error(s). (You already have the patient's full address on file.) There may be one error, more than one error, or no errors at all.

```
Anh Dang Tu, MD          Date _____
1145 Broadway
Anytown, USA
Pt. Name _____ Joan Neilsen _____
Address _____
Rx   Megace   40mg/ml
        1ml QID


Refills _____
        AD Tu
Substitution permitted      Dispense as written
```

1. Spot the error in the following prescription:

   _____

   A. Quantity missing
   B. Directions incomplete
   C. Strength missing
   D. Strength incorrect
   E. Dosage form incorrect

```
Anh Dang Tu, MD          Date _____
1145 Broadway
Anytown, USA
Pt. Name _____ Lili Ng _____
Address _____
Rx   tamoxifen   #30
        1 tab daily


Refills _____
        AD Tu
Substitution permitted      Dispense as written
```

2. Spot the error in the following prescription:

   _____

   A. Quantity missing
   B. Directions incorrect
   C. Strength missing
   D. Strength incorrect
   E. Dosage form incorrect

3. Give six pairs of drug names that have look-alike or sound-alike issues with drugs used to treat cancer.

DRUG NAME	LOOK-ALIKE OR SOUND-ALIKE DRUG

RESEARCH ACTIVITY

A new vaccine has been developed to decrease the risk of cancer linked to human papillomavirus (HPV). Access the National Library of Medicine's website (https://medlineplus.gov/hpv.html) and the Health Canada's website (https://www.canada.ca/en/public-health/services/diseases/human-papillomavirus-hpv.html) to answer the following questions about the HPV vaccine:

1. What is the trade name?

_____

_____

_____

_____

2. Who should get the vaccine?

_____

_____

_____

_____

_____

3. When is the vaccine contraindicated?

_____

_____

_____

_____

_____

4. What are its adverse effects?

_____

_____

_____

_____

_____

_____

5. How effective is the vaccine?

_____

_____

_____

_____

CASE STUDY

Joan is a 62-year-old female recently screened with a mammogram. Her doctor said her results may be a bit concerning and wants to run more tests. Joan has a sister who was diagnosed with breast cancer a few years back. Joan lives at home with her husband, has three children, and does not have a history of smoking or drinking.

1. Using information from Joan's history, what risk factors does she have for developing breast cancer?

_____

_____

_____

_____

2. List at least five factors that influence a patient's treatment options, including three that are specific to breast cancer.

_____

_____

_____

_____

Following a biopsy and other tests, the doctor has determined that the lump seen on Joan's mammogram is a malignant tumor. The cancer has not yet metastasized to other parts of Joan's body. She and her doctor decide to start with anastrozole, and trastuzumab.

3. Using your knowledge of these medications, explain what you know about the tumor's affinity for estrogen receptors and the expression of human epidermal growth factor receptor 2 (HER2).

_____

_____

_____

_____

4. Describe the mechanism of action of anastrozole.

_____

_____

_____

_____

32 Vaccines and Immunomodulators

TERMS AND DEFINITIONS

Match each term with the correct definition below.

A. Antigen
B. Cold chain
C. Conjugate vaccine
D. Immunomodulator
E. Immunosuppressant
F. Immunization
G. Inactivated killed vaccine
H. Live attenuated vaccine
I. Toxoid vaccine
J. Vaccine

1. A(n) _____ is a substance that prevents disease by taking advantage of your body's ability to make antibodies and release "killer" cells to disease.

2. The _____ is a set of safe handling practices that ensure vaccines and immunologic agents requiring refrigeration are maintained at a required temperature.

3. A(n) _____ links antigens or toxoids to polysaccharide or sugar molecules that certain bacteria use as a protective device to disguise themselves.

4. A drug that inhibits cell proliferation is known as a(n) _____.

5. A vaccine that stimulates the immune system to produce antibodies to a specific toxin that causes illness is called a(n) _____.

6. A(n) _____ is a deliberate, artificial exposure to disease to produce acquired immunity.

7. _____ is a living but weakened version of a disease.

8. _____ is a chemical agent that modifies the immune response or the functioning of the immune system.

9. A substance, usually a protein fragment, that causes an immune response is a(n) _____.

10. _____ provides less immunity than live vaccines but has fewer risks for vaccine-induced disease.

MULTIPLE CHOICE

1. Which of the following is **true** regarding inactivated killed vaccines? _____
   A. Inactivated killed vaccines can mutate to a virulent virus strain.
   B. Booster shots are usually needed for continued immunity.
   C. Inactivated killed vaccines produce greater immunity than live attenuated vaccines.
   D. MMR is an inactivated killed vaccine example.

2. Which of the following is **true** about the influenza vaccine? _____
   A. Flu vaccines are reformulated annually based on predictions of the virus epidemiologists believe will be most virulent.
   B. Influenza vaccine comes in an inactivated killed vaccine and a live attenuated vaccine form.
   C. The influenza vaccine is for those 6 months of age and older.
   D. All of the above

3. Select the **false** statement. Each time the cold chain is disrupted, _____.
   A. the effectiveness of the vaccine is reduced
   B. the loss of potency is cumulative
   C. the vaccine potency is unaffected
   D. the shelf life of the vaccine is reduced

4. Cold chain protocols for drugs should be established for all of the following *except* _____.
   A. receiving
   B. stocking
   C. storage
   D. transport
   E. administration

5. Which of the following reliably indicates the cold chain was broken during shipment?

   _____
   A. Thawed freezer packs
   B. Visible clumps after vaccine shaking
   C. A color change
   D. None of the above

6. Which of the following monoclonal antibody immunomodulators is used to prevent kidney transplant rejection? _____
   A. adalimumab
   B. basiliximab
   C. certolizumab
   D. daclizumab

7. Whereas vaccines boost the immune response, immunopharmacologic drugs such as cyclosporine _____.
   A. suppress cells of the immune system
   B. boost cells of the immune system
   C. have no effect on cells of the immune system

8. Cyclosporine _____.
   A. is derived from a bacterium
   B. suppresses rejection of organ transplants
   C. suppresses interferon-α
   D. has product formulations that are substitutable

9. Which drug is for mild to moderate chronic atopic dermatitis? _____
   A. basiliximab
   B. glatiramer
   C. tacrolimus
   D. temsirolimus

FILL IN THE BLANK: DRUG NAMES

1. What is the **brand name** for Hib conjugate vaccine? _____

2. What is the **generic name** for Boostrix and Adacel? _____

3. What is the **generic name** for Havrix? _____

4. What are the **brand names** for meningococcal group B conjugate vaccine? _____

5. What is the **generic name** for Engerix-B and Recombivax? _____

6. What is the **brand name** for pneumococcal 13-valent conjugate vaccine? _____

7. What is the **generic name** for Varivax? _____

8. What is the **brand name** for pneumococcal polysaccharide 23-polyvalent vaccine?

   _____

9. What is the **generic name** for RabAvert? _____

10. What is the **generic name** for Sandimmune and Neoral? _____

11. What is the **brand name** for sirolimus? _____

12. What is the **generic name** for Prograf and Protopic? _____

13. What is the **generic name** for Gammagard? _____

14. What is the **generic name** for CellCept? _____

15. What is the **brand name** for basiliximab? _____

16. What is the **generic name** for Thymoglobulin? _____

17. What is the **brand name** for daclizumab? _____

18. What is the **generic name** for WinRho SDF? _____

MATCHING

Patient education is an essential component of therapeutics. Select the **best** warning label to apply to the prescription vial given to patients taking the drugs listed.

A. TAKE ON AN EMPTY STOMACH

B. REFRIGERATE; DISCARD WITHIN 30 DAYS OF OPENING

C. SWALLOW CAPSULES WHOLE; DON'T CRUSH OR CHEW

D. PROTECT FROM LIGHT

1. _____ Rh$_o$[D] immune globulin

2. _____ cyclosporine caps

3. _____ sirolimus

4. _____ Prograf

TRUE OR FALSE

1. _____ A live attenuated vaccine can mutate to a virulent form of the disease.

2. _____ Cyclosporine oral liquid *nonmodified* (Sandimmune) is substitutable with cyclosporine oral liquid *modified* (Neoral, Gengraf).

3. _____ A common ending for monoclonal antibody immunomodulators is *-mab*.

4. _____ Dry powders are more sensitive to degradation. Therefore they are more likely to be affected by a breach in the cold chain than solutions.

5. _____ Rh$_o$[D] immune globulin is administered to pregnant women who are Rh (-) to prevent erythroblastosis fetalis.

6. _____ There is research currently being conducted on genetically engineered food as a delivery form for vaccines.

CRITICAL THINKING

The following hard copy is brought to your pharmacy for filling. Identify the prescription error(s). (You already have the patient's full address on file.) There may be one error, more than one error, or no errors at all.

Anh Dang Tu, MD Date _____
 1145 Broadway
 Anytown, USA
 	
 Pt. Name _____ Joan Neilsen _____
 Address _____
 ℞ *Sandimmune 100mg/ml*
      15mg/kg in 2 divided doses daily
 	
 Refills _____
     AD Tu _____
 Substitution permitted   Dispense as written
	1. Spot the error in the following prescription:
	
	 _____
	
	 A. Quantity missing
	 B. Directions incomplete
	 C. Strength missing
	 D. Strength incorrect
	 E. Dosage form incorrect

2. Give six pairs of drug names that have look-alike or sound-alike issues with drugs used to treat cancer.

DRUG NAME	LOOK-ALIKE OR SOUND-ALIKE DRUG

RESEARCH ACTIVITY

1. Pharmacists and pharmacy technicians play an important role in increasing community awareness of the importance of vaccination against vaccine-preventable illnesses. Search the Internet, and identify community initiatives run by pharmacies to increase public awareness.

_____

_____

_____

_____

_____

Cheryl has recently had a kidney transplant and brings new prescriptions to your pharmacy for prednisone, tacrolimus, and mycophenolate mofetil.

1. How should you educate Cheryl on tacrolimus and mycophenolate mofetil, especially with regard to meals?

_____

_____

_____

_____

2. Describe the mechanisms of action of tacrolimus and mycophenolate mofetil.

_____

_____

_____

_____

3. Immunosuppressant medications put patients at increased risk of infection. List some infections that Cheryl might have in the future.

_____

_____

_____

_____

Imagine that Cheryl's doctors chose belatacept (Nulojix) instead of tacrolimus to prevent transplant organ rejection.

4. Patients taking belatacept should not receive live attenuated vaccines. List at least four vaccines that would be contraindicated for Cheryl.

_____

_____

_____

_____

33 Treatment of Fungal Infections

TERMS AND DEFINITIONS

Match each term with the correct definition below.

A. Antifungal
B. *Candida*
C. Fungus (*pl.* fungi)
D. Mycosis
E. Onychomycosis
F. Ringworm
G. Vulvovaginal candidiasis

1. The general term for fungal infection is _____.

2. _____ is a fungal infection involving the fingernails or toenails.

3. A drug used to treat a fungal infection is called a(n) _____.

4. Another name for _____ is yeast vaginitis.

5. A(n) _____ is an organism similar to plants but lacking chlorophyll and capable of producing mycotic (fungal) infections.

6. Although its common name is "yeast," _____ is a type of fungus.

7. _____ is a group of tinea infections involving the body or scalp.

MULTIPLE CHOICE

1. Which condition cannot be treated over the counter (OTC)?

   _____
   A. Tinea pedis
   B. Onychomycosis
   C. Vulvovaginal candidiasis
   D. Jock itch

2. Which statement about ringworm is **false**?

   _____
   A. Infections are caused by a roundworm.
   B. Infections have a characteristic ringlike shape.
   C. Infections may be spread person to person.
   D. Infections may be spread animal to person.

3. Tinea capitis is a fungal infection located on the

   _____.
   A. torso
   B. fingernails
   C. scalp
   D. groin

4. Which of the following is *not* a mechanism of action of antifungal agents? _____
   A. Inhibiting antimetabolite activity
   B. Inhibiting fungal cell wall synthesis
   C. Fungal cell membrane destruction
   D. Interfering with nucleic acid synthesis

5. Select the drug that should *not* be taken concurrently with posaconazole. _____
   A. sertraline
   B. nitroglycerin SL
   C. cimetidine
   D. sucralfate

6. Common vaginal yeast infection risk factors include

   _____.
   A. broad-spectrum antibiotics, oral contraceptives, or hormone replacement therapy
   B. corticosteroids
   C. tight-fitting clothing and synthetic underwear
   D. All of the above

7. Which recommendation will *not* decrease the risk for recurrent athlete's foot infections? _____
   A. Keep feet clean and dry.
   B. Avoid walking barefoot across the floor of public facilities.
   C. Wear nylon socks.
   D. Use antifungal powders.

8. Select the antifungal drug that can be obtained without a prescription. _____
   A. Diflucan
   B. Sporanox
   C. clotrimazole
   D. posaconazole

9. Which antifungal should you take on an empty stomach? _____
   A. itraconazole
   B. voriconazole
   C. terbinafine
   D. griseofulvin

10. Select the antifungal that is indicated for prevention of athlete's foot. _____
    A. tolnaftate
    B. nystatin
    C. terbinafine
    D. griseofulvin
    E. miconazole

FILL IN THE BLANK: DRUG NAMES

1. What is the *brand name* for fluconazole? _____

2. What is the *generic name* for Lotrimin (United States) and Canesten (Canada)? _____

3. What is the *brand name* for itraconazole? _____

4. What is the *generic name* for Spectazole (United States)? _____

5. What is the *brand name* for oxiconazole (United States)? _____

6. What is the *generic name* for Nizoral? _____

7. What is the *brand name* for voriconazole? _____

8. What is the *generic name* for Monistat? _____

9. What is a *brand name* for nystatin? _____

10. What is the *generic name* for Noxafil (United States) and Posanol (Canada)? _____

11. What is the *brand name* for naftifine? _____

12. What is the *generic name* for Exelderm (United States)? _____

13. What is the *brand name* for tolnaftate? _____

14. What is the *generic name* for Terazol? _____

15. What is the *brand name* for caspofungin? _____

16. What is the *generic name* for Vagistat? _____

17. What are *brand names* for ciclopirox? _____

18. What is the *generic name* for Mentax (United States)? _____

19. What is the *generic name* for Gris-PEG? _____

20. What is the *generic name* for Lamisil? _____

21. What are **brand names** for undecylenic acid? _____

22. What is the **generic name** for Fungizone (Canada)? _____

23. What is the **generic name** for Natacyn? _____

24. What is the **brand name** for anidulafungin (United States)? _____

25. What is the **generic name** for Mycamine (United States)? _____

26. What is the **generic name** for Betadine? _____

MATCHING

Match the fungal infection to its location.

A. tinea cruris
B. tinea corporis
C. tinea unguium
D. thrush
E. tinea capitis

1. _____ mouth

2. _____ scalp

3. _____ groin

4. _____ nails

5. _____ body

MATCHING

Match the antifungal to its pharmacological class.

A. Allylamine
B. Echinocandin
C. Imidazole
D. Polyene
E. Thiocarbamate
F. Triazole

1. _____ voriconazole

2. _____ miconazole

3. _____ amphotericin B

4. _____ terbinafine

5. _____ micafungin

6. _____ tolnaftate

TRUE OR FALSE

1. _____ Tinea unguium is also known as onychomycosis.

2. _____ Griseofulvin is an orally administered drug used to treat onychomycosis.

3. _____ Echinocandins are formulated only for parenteral use.

4. _____ A common ending for allylamine antifungals is *-fungin*.

5. _____ Most fungal infections of the skin are caused by a group of fungi called dermatophytes.

6. _____ Women who take broad-spectrum antibiotics may develop a yeast infection.

7. _____ Diflucan is OTC in the United States.

8. _____ Nystatin, natamycin, and amphotericin B are all derived from the fungi-like bacteria.

9. _____ Griseofulvin should be taken with a high fat content meal.

10. _____ *Candida* thrives in cool, dry areas.

11. _____ Frequently removing and replacing artificial nails increases susceptibility to nail fungal infections.

CRITICAL THINKING

The following hard copies are brought to your pharmacy for filling. Identify the prescription error(s). (You already have the patient's full address on file.) There may be one error, more than one error, or no errors at all.

```
        Anh Dang Tu, MD       Date _____
          1145 Broadway
          Anytown, USA

Pt. Name _____ Joan Neilson _____
Address _____
Rx   Diflucan
     Take 2 tablets as a single dose    #2


Refills _____
       AD Tu                     _____
Substitution permitted        Dispense as written
```

1. Spot the error in the following prescription:

   _____

   A. Quantity missing
   B. Directions incomplete
   C. Strength missing
   D. Strength incorrect
   E. Dosage form incorrect

```
        Anh Dang Tu, MD       Date _____
          1145 Broadway
          Anytown, USA

Pt. Name _____ Lili Ng _____
Address _____
Rx   Noxafil 200mg/5ml
     200mg TID   SHAKE WELL


Refills _____
       AD Tu                     _____
Substitution permitted        Dispense as written
```

2. Spot the error in the following prescription:

   _____

   A. Quantity missing
   B. Directions incorrect
   C. Strength missing
   D. Strength incorrect
   E. Dosage form incorrect

3. Give six pairs of drug names that have look-alike or sound-alike issues with drugs used to treat fungal infections.

DRUG NAME	LOOK-ALIKE OR SOUND-ALIKE DRUG

Access the *Merck Manuals* website (http://www.merck.com/mmpe/sec10/ch125/ch125c.html) and Family Doctor's website (https://familydoctor.org/condition/nail-fungal-infections/) to conduct research on onychomycosis.

1. What are risk factors for development of this condition?

_____

_____

_____

_____

_____

2. Why is onychomycosis so difficult to treat?

_____

_____

_____

_____

_____

CASE STUDY

Brian comes to the pharmacy counter looking for a product to treat a rash on his foot. After asking a few questions, the pharmacist sees that the skin between Brian's toes is flaking, blistered, and red. Brian says it itches and burns. This started a couple of weeks ago after Brian began to take a kickboxing gym class, and the symptoms have become worse over the last few days. He says he has been showering at the gym before going home.

1. What infection does Brian probably have? Is this something that can be treated with OTC medications, or should the pharmacist refer Brian to his doctor?

_____

_____

_____

_____

2. List at least three topical creams available OTC (brand and generic names) the pharmacist can recommend to Brian.

_____

_____

_____

_____

3. How did Brian most likely acquire this infection? List at least five things Brian can do to prevent getting this infection again.

_____

_____

_____

_____

A few months later, Brian returns. He did not follow your advice for good foot hygiene. Now his toenails are thick, yellow, and crumbly. He asks, "Can I use the stuff I got last time" to treat his nails.

4. Can he treat this toenail fungal infection with OTC medications, or should the pharmacist refer Brian to his doctor?

_____

_____

_____

_____

34 Treatment of Pressure Injuries and Burns

TERMS AND DEFINITIONS

Match each term with the correct definition below.

A. Blister
B. Debridement
C. Pressure injury
D. Dehiscent wound
E. Eschar
F. First-degree burn
G. Fourth-degree burn
H. Full-thickness burn
I. Partial-thickness burns
J. Rule of palms
K. Rule of nines
L. Second-degree burn
M. Third-degree burn

1. A(n) _____ involves underlying muscles, fasciae, or bone.

2. _____ is blackened necrotic tissue of a pressure injury.

3. A "bedsore" is a type of _____.

4. A burn that involves deep epidermal layers and causes damage to the upper layers of dermis is called a(n) _____.

5. An injured area in which fluid collects below or within the epidermis as a result of a burn is called a(n) _____.

6. A(n) _____ causes minor discomfort and reddening of the skin.

7. A burn that is characterized by destruction of the epidermis and dermis is called a(n) _____.

8. First- and second-degree burns are also known as _____ ; in contrast, a third-degree burn is known as a(n) _____.

9. _____ is a surgical removal of foreign material and dead tissue from a wound to prevent infection and promote healing.

10. _____ is a formula for estimating the percentage of adult body surface covered by burns; it divides the body into 11 areas, each representing 9% of the body surface area.

11. _____ is a rule for estimating the extent of a burn surface area in which the palm size of the victim is about 1% of total body surface area.

12. A _____ is a wound that has reopened after it has been surgically closed.

1. Which advice is *not* given to a person who has

   caught on fire? _____
   A. Stop
   B. Drop
   C. Roll
   D. Run

2. One formula for estimating the percentage of adult body surface covered by burns is called the

   _____.
   A. Rule of fives
   B. Rule of sevens
   C. Rule of nines
   D. Rule of 12s

3. A third-degree burn _____.
   A. involves deep epidermal layers and causes damage to the upper layers of the dermis
   B. is characterized by destruction of the epidermis and dermis
   C. causes minor discomfort and reddening of the skin
   D. involves underlying muscles or bone

4. Which of the following is **false** about pressure

   injuries? _____
   A. Pressure injuries are "bedsores."
   B. To prevent these injuries, you should reposition an immobilized patient every 2 hours.
   C. The scale for assessing a patient's risk for developing pressure injuries runs from 1 to 4, with 4 representing the highest risk.
   D. Pressure injuries tend to form near bones close to the skin

5. Which answer correctly characterizes wound

   severity staging? _____
   A. Stage 1: wounds extend through skin involving underlying muscle, tendons, and bone.
   B. Stage 2: wounds have blisters and an exposed dermis.
   C. Stage 3: Infection is not a concern
   D. Stage 4: Skin is unbroken from a superficial wound

6. Debridement of dead tissue is accomplished by applying all of the following *except*

   _____.
   A. collagenase
   B. hydrocortisone
   C. papain and urea
   D. Granulex

7. The most commonly used topical medicine for the

   treatment of burns is _____.
   A. erythromycin ointment
   B. silver sulfadiazine cream
   C. butter
   D. hydrocortisone cream

8. Which is a potential burn complication?

   _____
   A. Scarring
   B. Bone and joint problems
   C. Pneumonia
   D. Infection
   E. All of the above

9. The most common adverse effect of mafenide is

   _____.
   A. itchiness
   B. burning
   C. coldness
   D. dry skin

FILL IN THE BLANK: DRUG NAMES

1. What is a **brand name** for bacitracin? _____

2. What is the **generic name** for Santyl? _____

3. What is the **generic name** for Polysporin? _____

4. What are the **brand names** for mupirocin? _____

5. What is the *generic name* for Silvadene (United States) and Flamazine (Canada)?

   _____

6. What is the *brand name* for mafenide? _____

7. What is the *generic name* for Betadine? _____

TRUE OR FALSE

1. _____ According to the rule of palms, a burn victim's palm size is equivalent to about 5% of total body surface area.

2. _____ There are three categories of burns (first, second, and third degree).

3. _____ An alternative name for first- and second-degree burns is partial-thickness burns.

4. _____ In treating pressure injuries, one should remove necrotic tissue from the wound.

5. _____ Two common complications of burns are infection and edema.

6. _____ Fourth-degree burns result in a patient insensitive to pain just after injury.

CRITICAL THINKING

The following hard copies are brought to your pharmacy for filling. Identify the prescription error(s). (You already have the patient's full address on file.) There may be one error, more than one error, or no errors at all.

Anh Dang Tu, MD   Date _____
1145 Broadway
Anytown, USA

Pt. Name _____ Joan Neilson _____
Address _____

℞ Silver sulfadiazine cream
   Apply once or twice daily with sterile-gloved hand

Refills _____

_____ AD Tu _____   _____
Substitution permitted   Dispense as written

---

1. Spot the error in the following prescription:

   _____

   A. Quantity missing
   B. Directions incomplete
   C. Strength missing
   D. Strength incorrect
   E. Dosage form incorrect

Anh Dang Tu, MD   Date _____
1145 Broadway
Anytown, USA

Pt. Name _____ Lili Ng _____
Address _____

℞ Santyl ointment   250 units/Gm
   apply once daily

Refills _____

_____ AD Tu _____   _____
Substitution permitted   Dispense as written

---

2. Spot the error in the following prescription:

   _____

   A. Quantity missing
   B. Directions incorrect
   C. Strength missing
   D. Strength incorrect
   E. Dosage form incorrect

3. Give four pairs of drug names that have look-alike or sound-alike issues with drugs used to treat wounds.

DRUG NAME	LOOK-ALIKE OR SOUND-ALIKE DRUG

RESEARCH ACTIVITY

1. Some hospital pharmacies raise maggots. Conduct an Internet search to discover the current use of maggots in medicine, and write a paragraph describing this process.

_____

_____

_____

_____

_____

CASE STUDY

Gene is an elderly male living at home with diabetes. He's independent, but his daughter comes into your pharmacy looking for a product to help a sore on Gene's hip. Gene's health has declined over the last few months. He is not very mobile and spends most days in his recliner. He has also not been eating well as of late. You ask Gene's daughter to take a picture of the sore, and she brings it to you. You see a nickel-sized broken blister surrounded by redness on his hip.

1. What stage characterizes Gene's wound? Should the pharmacist instruct the daughter to seek medical assistance immediately, or can this be treated at home?

_____

_____

_____

_____

2. The goal of care is to cover, protect, and clean the area. List at least four dressing types that would be appropriate to cover and protect Gene's wound.

_____

_____

_____

_____

3. What other measures can Gene and his daughter take to heal his wound and to prevent further pressure injuries?

_____

_____

_____

_____

4. What is the biggest concern with Stage 3 and 4 wounds?

_____

_____

_____

_____

5. List three different products a wound care specialist could choose for debridement to slough off necrotic tissue from the pressure injury.

_____

_____

_____

_____

35 Treatment of Acne

TERMS AND DEFINITIONS

Match each term with the correct definition below.

A. Acne
B. Acne vulgaris
C. Blackhead
D. Comedones
E. Cysts
F. Keratolytic
G. Milia
H. Nodule
I. Papule
J. Pustule
K. Whitehead

1. A(n) _____ agent is a peeling agent.

2. A(n) _____ is a large, inflamed lesion and may be superficial or deep.

3. _____ is a condition that occurs as a result of the action of hormones and other substances on the skin's oil glands and hair follicles.

4. A(n) _____ contains sebum and bacteria that have become trapped in the hair follicle and move to the surface.

5. An obstructed follicle that becomes inflamed is called a(n)

   _____.

6. _____ are tiny little bumps that occur when normally sloughed skin cells get trapped in small pockets on the surface of the skin.

7. A pimple that contains trapped sebum and bacteria and stays below the

   skin surface is called a(n) _____.

8. _____ are deep, painful pus-filled lesions that can cause scarring.

9. The most characteristic sign of acne is enlarged, plugged hair follicles or

   _____.

10. A large, painful solid lesion lodged deep in the skin is called a(n)

    _____.

11. _____ is the most common form of acne.

MULTIPLE CHOICE

1. Factors that make acne worse include all of the
   following *except* _____.
   A. changing hormone levels in adolescence
   B. grease encountered in the work environment
   C. cosmetics
   D. chocolate
   E. stress

2. Drugs that can cause acne include all of the following
   except _____ .
   A. lithium
   B. penicillin
   C. prednisone
   D. phenytoin

3. What is the goal of acne treatment?
   _____
   A. Heal existing lesions
   B. Stop new lesion formation
   C. Prevent scarring
   D. Reduce psychological stress
   E. All of the above

4. Acne is treated with the administration of all of the
   following *except* _____.
   A. antibiotics
   B. keratolytics
   C. topical corticosteroids
   D. oral contraceptives

5. Which statement about isotretinoin is **false**?
   _____
   A. Women taking isotretinoin must use birth control
      for 1 month prior to treatment, throughout the
      duration of treatment, and for 1 month after
      stopping treatment.
   B. Isotretinoin is taken once or twice daily, orally,
      with food.
   C. Baseline kidney function tests are taken before
      starting treatment.
   D. Isotretinoin decreases the size and output of
      sebaceous glands.

6. In the United States, prescribers, pharmacies, and
   patients are required to register in the FDA iPLEDGE
   program as a condition for use of _____
   to minimize risks of birth defects.
   A. minocycline
   B. erythromycin
   C. isotretinoin
   D. tetracycline

7. Which topical medication is the most effective and
   widely used nonprescription medication available for
   noninflammatory acne?
   _____
   A. clindamycin gel
   B. erythromycin solution
   C. tazarotene
   D. benzoyl peroxide

8. _____ works by killing the bacteria that
   infect pores.
   A. Tazarotene
   B. Azelaic acid
   C. Adapalene
   D. Tretinoin

9. Which oral antibiotic is a first-line therapy for
   Propionibacterium acnes (P. acnes)?
   _____
   A. doxycycline
   B. erythromycin
   C. clindamycin
   D. amoxicillin

FILL IN THE BLANK: DRUG NAMES

1. What are the **brand names** for doxycycline hyclate? _____

2. What is the **generic name** for PanOxyl? _____

3. What is the **generic name** for Epiduo? _____

4. What is the **brand name** for adapalene? _____

5. What is the *generic name* for Aczone? _____

6. What is the *generic name* for Azelex (United States) and Finacea (Canada)? _____

7. What is the *brand name* for benzoyl peroxide and erythromycin? _____

8. What is the *brand name* for alitretinoin? _____

9. What is the *brand name* for tazarotene? _____

10. What is the *generic name* for Benzaclin? _____

11. What is the *generic name* for Accutane? _____

12. What is the *generic name* for Minocin? _____

13. What is the *generic name* for Renova and Retin-A? _____

14. What is the *generic name* for Ziana (United States)? _____

MATCHING

Patient education is an essential component of therapeutics. Select the **best** warning label to apply to the prescription vial given to patients taking the drugs listed.

A. AVOID PREGNANCY

B. BLEACHING AGENT—AVOID
   CONTACT WITH FABRIC
   AND HAIR

C. MAY CAUSE SENSITIVITY
   TO SUNLIGHT

D. AVOID TAKING ANTACIDS,
   IRON, AND DAIRY
   PRODUCTS

1. _____ Retin-A 0.025%

2. _____ minocycline 100 mg

3. _____ benzoyl peroxide 10%

4. _____ Accutane 20 mg

TRUE OR FALSE

1. _____ Pilosebaceous units consist of a sebaceous gland connected to a hair follicle.

2. _____ A blackhead is a closed comedone.

3. _____ Acne vulgaris occurs most frequently in the adolescent years.

4. _____ Benzoyl peroxide may cause dry skin and redness.

5. _____ Blackheads appear black because of changes in sebum as it is exposed to air.

6. _____ *Propionibacterium* is a bacterium that causes acne.

7. _____ Milia are a serious skin condition in newborns that should be treated with medications.

8. _____ It often takes 6 to 8 weeks before oral antibiotics show evidence of improving acne.

CRITICAL THINKING

The following hard copies are brought to your pharmacy for filling. Identify the prescription error(s). (You already have the patient's full address on file.) There may be one error, more than one error, or no errors at all.

Anh Dang Tu, MD   Date _____
1145 Broadway
Anytown, USA

Pt. Name _____ John Neilson _____
Address _____
℞   Retin-A gel   45Gm
       apply nightly

Refills _____
_____ AD Tu
Substitution permitted   Dispense as written

---

1. Spot the error in the following prescription:

   _____

   A. Quantity missing
   B. Directions incomplete
   C. Strength missing
   D. Strength incorrect
   E. Dosage form incorrect

Anh Dang Tu, MD   Date _____
1145 Broadway
Anytown, USA

Pt. Name _____ Lili Newell _____
Address _____
℞   Minocycline 100mg BID

Refills _____
_____ AD Tu
Substitution permitted   Dispense as written

---

2. Spot the error in the following prescription:

   _____

   A. Quantity missing
   B. Directions incorrect
   C. Strength missing
   D. Strength incorrect
   E. Dosage form incorrect

---

3. Give six pairs of drug names that have look-alike or sound-alike issues with drugs used to treat acne.

DRUG NAME	LOOK-ALIKE OR SOUND-ALIKE DRUG

4. You are asked to compound clindamycin 2% solution from clindamycin 75-mg capsules and commercially prepared clindamycin 1% solution (60 mL). How many capsules will you need to add to the commercially prepared solution? Please show your calculations.

_____

_____

_____

_____

RESEARCH ACTIVITY

1. Severe acne can be disfiguring. Access the National Library of Medicine's website (http://www.nlm.nih.gov/medlineplus/acne.html#cat11) and other websites to learn more about acne. Write a paragraph about the social impact of acne.

_____

_____

_____

_____

CASE STUDY

A teenage girl and her mother approach a pharmacy checkout counter. The girl looks embarrassed as the mother says they are looking for acne treatment. The mother says, "I told her to stop eating junk food, but her breakouts are getting worse."

1. Is junk food contributing to acne? List at least four factors that can worsen acne.

_____

_____

_____

2. Describe the four different types of inflammatory acne lesions associated with breakouts.

_____

_____

_____

_____

After examining the girl's condition, the pharmacist determines that she has mild acne. He recommends that she gently wash her face twice daily with warm water and a mild soap. He then takes her to the acne area in the over-the-counter section to help her select a medication to treat and prevent future breakouts. There are many options, but the pharmacist explains that they all contain the same active ingredient.

3. Which is the most effective and widely used nonprescription medication for acne?

_____

_____

_____

_____

4. Describe the mechanism of action of benzoyl peroxide.

_____

_____

_____

5. What is an important point the pharmacist should tell the mother and daughter about products containing benzoyl peroxide?

_____

_____

_____

_____

36 Treatment of Atopic Dermatitis and Psoriasis

TERMS AND DEFINITIONS

Match each term with the correct definition below.

A. Atopic dermatitis
B. Cutaneous
C. Dermatitis
D. Eczema
E. Phototherapy
F. Psoriasis
G. Plaque psoriasis

1. The term used to describe inflammation of the skin is _____.

2. _____ is a treatment for atopic dermatitis that involves exposing the skin to ultraviolet A or B light waves.

3. A chronic disease of the skin, _____ is characterized by itchy red patches covered with silvery scales.

4. _____is a chronic inflammatory condition that affects the skin.

5. A general term used to describe several types of inflammation of the skin is _____.

6. _____ is a term that means pertaining to the skin.

7. _____ is the most common form of psoriasis.

MULTIPLE CHOICE

1. Irritants that aggravate the skin of persons with

   atopic dermatitis are _____.
   A. cotton and silk
   B. perfumes and cosmetics
   C. rice and potatoes
   D. cleaning solvents and detergents
   E. B and D

2. Psoriatic patches are typically found in all of the

   regions *except* _____.
   A. neck
   B. face
   C. elbows
   D. genitals
   E. hands and feet

3. Which advice would *not* be given to a person with

   eczema? _____.
   A. Avoid wearing wool or clothing that feels "scratchy."
   B. Increase humidity in the household environment.
   C. Apply moisturizers and lotion to the skin.
   D. Take hot baths.

4. Of the following, the most potent corticosteroid

   classification is _____.
   A. class I
   B. class II
   C. class III
   D. class IV
   E. class V

5. Select the corticosteroid that is in the least potent

   category. _____
   A. clobetasol
   B. betamethasone dipropionate (optimized)
   C. hydrocortisone base cream
   D. halobetasol propionate
   E. fluocinonide

6. Which of the following adverse effects is not linked

   to topical use of corticosteroids? _____
   A. thinning of the skin
   B. Cushing's syndrome
   C. stretch marks (striae)
   D. spider veins
   E. acne

7. Select the drug that is indicated for the treatment of

   severe psoriasis and arthritis. _____
   A. cyclosporine
   B. azathioprine
   C. methotrexate
   D. calcipotriene

8. Which of the following correctly describes the
   mechanism of action of topical corticosteroids?

   _____
   A. Corticosteroids decrease redness, swelling, and
      inflammation by reducing the number of
      inflammatory cells.
   B. Corticosteroids increase cell permeability to T
      lymphocytes and eosinophils.
   C. Corticosteroids increase cytokine release.
   D. Topical corticosteroids cause vasodilation.

9. The FDA and Health Canada require manufacturers
   to include a Black Box warning in the package

   insert for _____, describing the
   increased risks for cancer.
   A. Dermatop-E and Dovonex
   B. Cutivate and Ultravate
   C. methotrexate and Enbrel
   D. pimecrolimus and tacrolimus

10. Dovonex is a synthetic analog of _____.
    A. vitamin A
    B. vitamin B
    C. vitamin C
    D. vitamin D

FILL IN THE BLANK: DRUG NAMES

1. What is a **brand name** for betamethasone dipropionate? _____

2. What is the **generic name** for Soriatane? _____

3. What is the **generic name** for Luxiq (United States) and Valisone-G (Canada)? _____

4. What is the **brand name** for desoximetasone? _____

5. What is the **generic name** for ApexiCon E? _____

6. What are **brand names** for fluocinolone acetonide? _____

7. What is the **generic name** for Clobex? _____

8. What is the **brand name** for fluticasone? _____

9. What is the **generic name** for DesOwen (United States)? _____

10. What is the **brand name** for halcinonide? _____

11. What is the **generic name** for Tazorac? _____

12. What is the **brand name** for halobetasol? _____

13. What is the **brand name** for clocortolone? _____

14. What is the **brand name** for hydrocortisone valerate (Canada)? _____

15. What is the **generic name** for Lidex? _____

16. What is the **brand name** for prednicarbate? _____

17. What is the **generic name** for Cordran? _____

18. What is the **brand name** for pimecrolimus? _____

19. What is the **generic name** for Locoid (United States)? _____

20. What is the **brand name** for tacrolimus? _____

21. What is the **generic name** for Elocon (United States) and Elocom (Canada)? _____

22. What is the **brand name** for calcipotriene (United States) and calcipotriol (Canada)?

    _____

23. What is the **generic name** for Vectical (United States) and Silkis (Canada)? _____

24. What are **brand names** for methoxsalen? _____

25. What is the **generic name** for Taclonex (United States) and Dovobet (Canada)? _____

26. What are **brand names** for infliximab? _____

27. What is the **generic name** for Neoral? _____

28. What is the **brand name** for etanercept? _____

29. What is the **generic name** for Stelara? _____

30. What is the **generic name** for Otezla? _____

MATCHING

Match each drug to its pharmacological classification.

A. furanocoumarins
B. corticosteroid
C. vitamin D analog
D. calcineurin inhibitor
E. immunosuppressants

1. _____ Dovonex

2. _____ methotrexate

3. _____ mometasone

4. _____ Elidel

5. _____ Oxsoralen-Ultra

MATCHING

Patient education is an essential component of therapeutics. Select the **best** warning label to apply to the prescription container given to patients taking the drugs listed.

A. AVOID PROLONGED EXPOSURE TO SUNLIGHT
B. REFRIGERATE; DO NOT FREEZE
C. SWALLOW WHOLE; DON'T CRUSH OR CHEW
D. AVOID CONTACT WITH FACE
E. AVOID SUN EXPOSURE FOR 24 HOURS BEFORE AND 48 HOURS AFTER TREATMENT

1. _____ Elidel

2. _____ methoxsalen

3. _____ apremilast

4. _____ Enbrel

5. _____ Taclonex

TRUE OR FALSE

1. _____ Stress and dry skin may aggravate psoriasis.

2. _____ It is uncommon for eczema that has gone into remission in childhood to return with the onset of puberty.

3. _____ Corticosteroids are categorized into five potency categories.

4. _____ Topical corticosteroids possess antiinflammatory and immunosuppressive properties.

5. _____ Phototherapy involves exposing the skin to ultraviolet A, B, and C light waves.

6. _____ The vehicle (base) in which the corticosteroid is suspended has no influence on potency.

7. _____ Eczema is a specific type of atopic dermatitis.

8. _____ Phototherapy can prematurely age skin and increase patients' skin cancer risk.

9. _____ Atopic dermatitis is believed to be an autoimmune disease.

10. _____ Elidel and Protopic are topical agents for plaque psoriasis.

CRITICAL THINKING

The following hard copy is brought to your pharmacy for filling. Identify the prescription error(s). (You already have the patient's full address on file.) There may be one error, more than one error, or no errors at all.

```
        Anh Dang Tu, MD      Date _____
          1145 Broadway
          Anytown, USA

Pt. Name _____ Joan Neilson _____
Address _____
Rx   triancinolone 0.025%     15Gm
     apply sparingly to affected area TID



Refills _____

_____ AD Tu _____          _____
Substitution permitted        Dispense as written
```

1. Spot the error in the following prescription:

   _____

   A. Quantity missing
   B. Directions incomplete
   C. Strength missing
   D. Strength incorrect
   E. Dosage form missing

2. Give six pairs of drug names that have look-alike or sound-alike issues with drugs used to treat eczema and psoriasis.

DRUG NAME	LOOK-ALIKE OR SOUND-ALIKE DRUG

RESEARCH ACTIVITY

1. Review Chapter 1 and research the Internet to learn about drug product formulation. Write a paragraph explaining why the potency of corticosteroids is influenced by the vehicle in which the drug is mixed.

_____

_____

_____

_____

CASE STUDY

Martha is a pharmacy patient who comes to the counter and asks for "the creams for my skin condition." You notice that Martha has thick, silvery, scaly patches on her hands and elbows. You examine her medication profile and fill her prescriptions for betamethasone cream and Dovonex cream.

1. Using your understanding of Martha's medications and symptoms, what kind of skin condition do you think she has?

_____

_____

_____

_____

2. List at least four factors that can exacerbate symptoms of atopic dermatitis and psoriasis.

_____

_____

_____

_____

Next month, Martha returns to the pharmacy after a visit with her dermatologist. She hands you a Humira prescription.

3. Adalimumab (Humira) is a biologic monoclonal antibody. What is the target of adalimumab?

_____

_____

_____

_____

4. List some adverse effects associated with adalimumab.

_____

_____

_____

_____

5. Identify another biologic agent with the same target that Martha's doctor could have selected to treat her condition.

_____

_____

_____

_____

37 Treatment of Lice and Scabies

TERMS AND DEFINITIONS

Match each term with the correct definition below.

A. Lice
B. Nits
C. Nymph
D. Ovicidal
E. Parasite
F. Pediculicide
G. Scabies
H. Scabicide

1. An organism that benefits by living in, with, or on another organism is called a _____.

2. A(n) _____ is a drug that kills _____, a parasitic mite that causes infection.

3. A drug that is _____ is able to kill the eggs of lice.

4. Another name for head lice eggs is _____.

5. A drug that kills lice is called a(n) _____.

6. _____ are a group of parasites that can live on the body, scalp, or genital area of humans.

7. The term used to describe a baby louse is _____.

MULTIPLE CHOICE

1. Which parasite is *not* a louse? _____
   A. *Pediculus humanus capitis*
   B. *Sarcoptes scabiei*
   C. *Pediculus humanus corporis*
   D. *Phthirus pubis*

2. _____ is a parasitic infection classified as a sexually transmitted infection (STI).
   A. *Pediculus humanus capitis*
   B. scabies
   C. *Pediculus humanus corporis*
   D. *Phthirus pubis*

3. Pharmacy technicians should apply the warning label _____ to prescription vials containing lindane shampoo.
   A. SHAKE WELL
   B. DILUTE BEFORE USE
   C. FOR EXTERNAL USE ONLY
   D. APPLY SPARINGLY

4. Which warning should be given to persons receiving a prescription for malathion? _____
   A. AVOID OPEN FLAMES (e.g., LIT CIGARETTES, CIGARS, AND PIPES)
   B. MAY STAIN CLOTHING AND HAIR
   C. MAY BLEACH CLOTHING AND HAIR
   D. DILUTE BEFORE USE

5. Select the drug for which the FDA requires manufacturers to place a Black Box warning in the package insert. _____
   A. lindane
   B. permethrins
   C. pyrethrins
   D. crotamiton

6. Lindane is _____.
   A. nephrotoxic
   B. neurotoxic
   C. hepatotoxic
   D. ototoxic

7. Spinosad works by _____.
   A. paralyzing the parasites' CNS with an acetylcholine accumulation
   B. dissolving the exoskeleton of a louse
   C. asphyxiating lice
   D. producing neuronal excitation in lice, resulting in paralysis and death

8. Which of the following statements about body lice is **false**? _____
   A. Body lice infestations are caused by the parasite *Pediculus humanus corporis*.
   B. Adult body lice can survive away from a human host for 30 days.
   C. Body lice infestations are a serious public health concern.
   D. Body lice may cause epidemics of typhus and louse-borne relapsing fever.

9. In which environmental conditions does scabies thrive? _____
   A. dense populations such as in prisons and nursing homes
   B. warm environment
   C. moist environment
   D. arid environment
   E. scarcely populated environment

10. Strategies to prevent lice reinfestation include all of the following *except* _____.
    A. Treat all household members.
    B. Wash clothing, linens, and bedding in hot water.
    C. Throw away toys, clothing, and bedding that cannot be washed.
    D. Use a nit comb to remove eggs.

FILL IN THE BLANK: DRUG NAMES

1. What is the *generic name* for Ovide (United States)? _____

2. What is the *brand name* for crotamiton? _____

3. What is the *generic name* for Elimite Cream and Nix? _____

4. What is the *generic name* for RID (United States) and R&C (Canada)? _____

5. What is the *brand name* for benzyl alcohol? _____

6. What is the *generic name* for Sklice? _____

7. What is the *generic name* for Natroba? _____

TRUE OR FALSE

1. _____ Treatment of head lice requires shaving the head.

2. _____ Malathion was withdrawn from the market in Canada but is still available in the United States.

3. _____ Head lice most commonly affect children aged 3 to 11 years.

4. _____ Head lice infestation is caused by poor hygiene.

5. _____ Individuals *cannot* get pubic lice from sitting on public toilet seats.

6. _____ Permethrin is approved for the treatment of head lice, body lice, and pubic lice.

7. _____ Permethrin is ovicidal (kills eggs), but pyrethrins are not.

8. _____ Ivermectin is safe to use in pregnant women.

9. _____ Permethrins and pyrethrins may be obtained only by prescription.

10. _____ Lindane is a first-line therapy for treating scabies.

CRITICAL THINKING

The following hard copy is brought to your pharmacy for filling. Identify the prescription error(s). (You already have the patient's full address on file.) There may be one error, more than one error, or no errors at all.

```
┌─────────────────────────────────────────────┐
│         Anh Dang Tu, MD      Date _____    │
│            1145 Broadway                       │
│            Anytown, USA                         │
│                                                 │
│  Pt. Name _____ Julie Nelson _____   │
│  Address _____ │
│  ℞  crotamiton 10% cream                        │
│     Apply after bathing to the skin over the    │
│     entire body from the chin to the toes.      │
│     Repeat in 24 hours. Bathe 48 hours AFTER    │
│     second dose.                                │
│  Refills _____                                 │
│  _____ AD Tu _____                       │
│  Substitution permitted      Dispense as written│
└─────────────────────────────────────────────┘
```

1. Spot the error in the following prescription:

   _____

   A. Quantity missing

   B. Directions incomplete

   C. Strength missing

   D. Strength incorrect

   E. Dosage form missing

2. Give one pair of drug names that have look-alike or sound-alike issues with drugs used to treat lice and scabies.

DRUG NAME	LOOK-ALIKE OR SOUND-ALIKE DRUG

RESEARCH ACTIVITY

1. Conduct an Internet search on the use of antiparasitic agents and antibiotics in agriculture. Write a paragraph explaining how their use may affect the treatment of infection in humans.

   _____

   _____

   _____

   _____

   _____

CASE STUDY

Lisa is a mother to two young children. She comes to your pharmacy counter in a panic because there is a lice outbreak at her children's daycare center. She is on her way home from work and has not had a chance to determine whether her children have an active case, but she wants to pick up a product to treat all of her family members.

1. What are two options for treating lice that are available over the counter in the United States?

   _____

   _____

   _____

   _____

2. Lisa chooses to purchase Nix. What are two important points that would help Lisa most effectively treat and remove the lice?

_____

_____

_____

_____

3. In addition to treating all family members, list five strategies to help prevent lice reinfestation in Lisa's home.

_____

_____

_____

_____

Lisa returns to your pharmacy 3 weeks later. She is upset because she treated all of her family members with Nix and followed all of the pharmacist's instructions, but she found a louse and several nits in her daughter's hair. She heard from a friend that there is a problem with "super lice."

4. Explain the problem of drug resistance in relationship to pediculicides.

_____

_____

_____

_____

Lisa returns from her pediatrician's office with a prescription for Sklice 0.5% solution.

5. Lisa's daughter is 6 years old and weighs 44 lbs. Is Sklice safe to use on Lisa's daughter?

_____

_____

_____

_____

6. Describe the mechanism of action of ivermectin.

_____

_____

_____

_____